Don't diet; change your habits

Don't diet; change your habits

Don't diet; change your habits

Copyright © 2018 *Carole St-Laurent a.k.a* Kina Diamond

Published by Fat Cat Publishing

Book ISBN color: 978-1-9994769-5-3

Book ISBN Black and white: 978-1-9994769-0-8

eBook ISBN: 978-1-9994769-1-5

Disclaimer

All the material contained in this book is provided for educational and informational purposes only. No responsibility can be taken for any results or outcomes resulting from the use of this material.

While every attempt has been made to provide information that is both accurate and effective, the author does not assume any responsibility for the accuracy or use/misuse of this information.

Use this information at your own will.

All pictures are cc from pixabay.com

Cover design by Carole St-Laurent

Don't diet; change your habits

Don't diet; change your habits

Contents

Don't diet; change your habits

Don't diet; change your habits

Introduction

Imagine...

Keeping up with your kids?

Living a long, healthy life?

Feeling sexy, confident, and vibrant?

This guide is conveyed with refreshing humor and honesty, this common-sense approach to weight loss will have you wonder why everybody isn't applying the methods suggested in this no-nonsense, straight forward health and weight loss guide.

This handbook is not a manual for people looking for quick fixes, rapid weight loss, nor is it a cleansing diet.

It is, more importantly, a lifestyle change that can be tweaked to every personal situation. Whether you are a chronic dieter, an emotional eater, or you just love food.

If getting up from the floor is problematic...

If you have a tough time tying your shoes...

If you are out of breath after playing with your kids...

If you view walking up-stairs as a treacherous terrain...

If you feel sluggish all the time...

This easy to understand weight loss guide will provide you with much-needed simplicity on a topic that gets muddled with unnecessary complexity.

Incidentally, there are lots of ways to lose weight but few to keep it off in a healthy, sustainable manner such as demonstrated in this health guide.

In short, this book offers straight forward methods to lose weight and get your health back on track.

So, get ready to welcome a new and improved you.

Look good and feel it!

Don't diet; change your habits

A journey of the mind and body

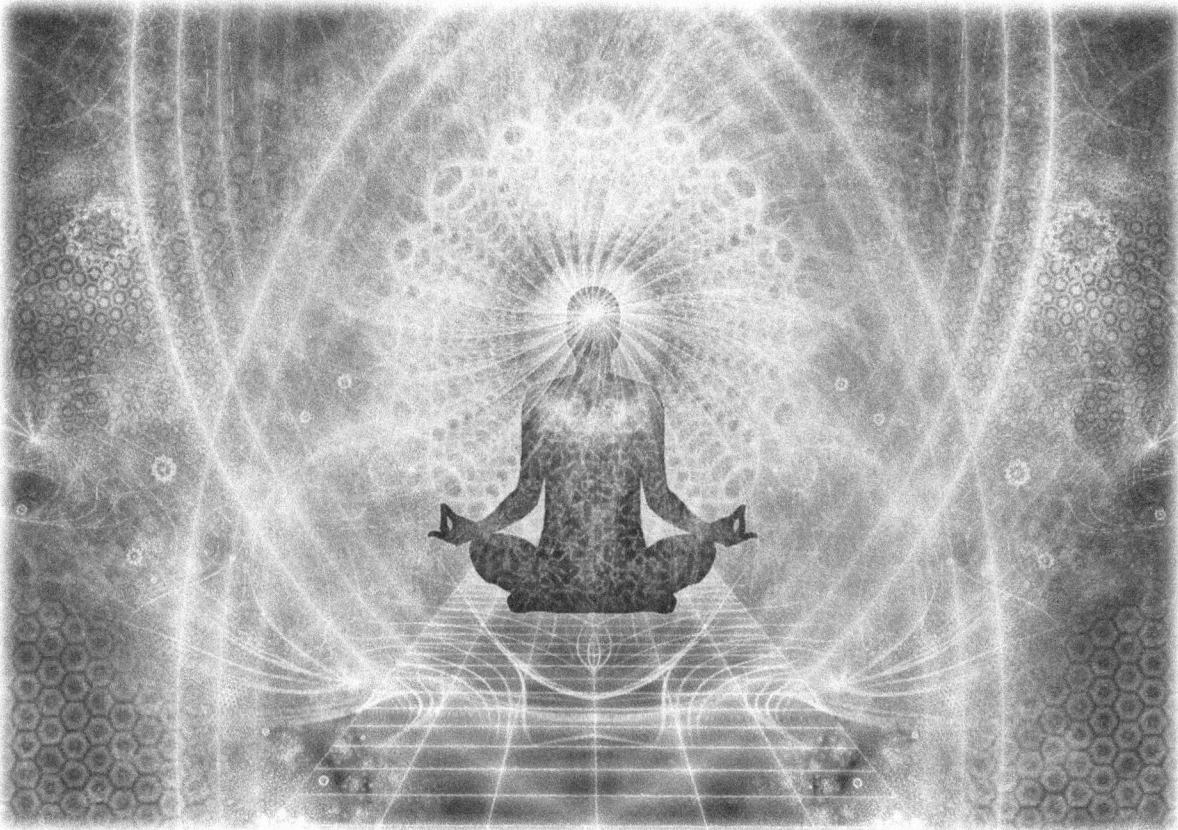

Welcome to "**Don't diet; change your habits**."

Before we begin, some things must be explained and well understood.

You should not want to lose weight to fit society's beauty standards. You should aim to get healthy, which will, in turn, make you lose weight.

You need to be mentally ready to lose weight.

Before you start losing weight, you must love and appreciate your body for the extraordinary organic apparatus that it is.

It is essential that you also be very appreciative of your body **as** it loses weight.

Because your body will be working hard for you, it will consume your extra fat. It will also reshape entirely. That is something!

Likewise, if you give your body the nutrients that it needs, the love that it desires, and the appreciation that it craves, it will metamorphose itself into a healthy, sexy body for you.

Consequently, what it all means is that you must stop hating your body.

So many women think negatively about their self-image.

They only see the bulging belly, the love handles, the double chin, the protruding butt and so on.

They feel ugly and hopeless as they fixate on their excess fat.

They look at thin, healthy women as being so perfect and better than they are.

They believe that thin women have some kind of advantage, a superpower that gives THEM the ability to lose weight and stay fit.

However, the fact is that they are not any different than you. You **are** as able and formidable as those women are.

You don't have fat genes, you are not born to stay this way, you most certainly are not hopeless, and you **CAN** take charge of your health to look and feel amazing.

Most importantly, you need to start this weight loss journey from a place of **self-love**.

If you don't change this attitude, even once the fat is gone, you will still have a negative self-image.

You will never feel beautiful enough.

Accept yourself first so that you can then improve.

Don't forget, your mind and your body are your allies. Together you are powerful, a force to be reckoned with.

So, you see, you are not alone in all of this.

Besides the hundreds of thousands of women that are going through the exact same emotional struggle as you are, you also have your mind and body to support you.

In fact, you are actually 3 entities working in synergy for the same healthy goal.

I can see you frowning right now, thinking, mind and body, those are 2 entities. Here is why you are 3...

First, there is the conscious you, also called the Ego, then the unconscious "the mind" and the body. You are all working together towards 1 goal, health.

If there is no harmony between the 3, there is conflict which results in physical and psychological imbalance.

In many of us, that imbalance manifests itself in disease and FAT.

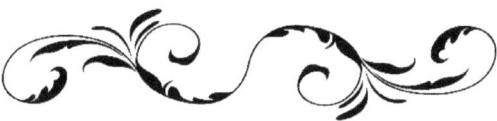

Unlike most weight loss books and programs which usually prone fast and easy weight loss. We realistically prepare you for your journey back to health.

One of the essential ingredients you must first acquire to lose weight is belief — first, you have to believe that you have what it takes to lose weight.

If you assume that it's in your family, that you are born to be fat or that you cannot lose weight, you make it a self-fulfilling prophecy.

Decidedly, there **will** be times when you will slip up. That is normal, and you should not feel defeated.

Remember that when pursuing any worthy goal, the journey is never linear.

It's often filled with setbacks, slip-ups, mistakes, etc.

But remember that every setback makes way for success.

Don't give up and go eating everything in sight, just because you slipped-up after work and ate a big pizza slice.

When you slip up on your diet, acknowledge your mistake and strive not to make any more. Don't throw in the towel just because of 1 faux pas.

Anyways, if for the next few days you are reasonable and eat sensibly, this small slip-up will be insignificant.

If you give up and fall back into your old eating routine of unhealthy food, you are guaranteed to regain what you worked so hard to lose and faster than you can say apple-crumble-delight.

Slipping-up once is NOT a sign of failure. Acknowledge your present mistake, correct it, avoid future indiscretion, and KEEP MOVING FORWARD.

That is the only way to succeed.

Trust that you're in control of your body, and you can change for the better if you know how to, and this health and weight loss guide will show you different options that are at your reach.

Follow it, and you will attain your desired weight.

Not only will you finally look the way you always wanted to. You will feel so much more energetic. You will gain strength and have a sense of accomplishment that just can't be described.

Chapter 1

The ugly truth

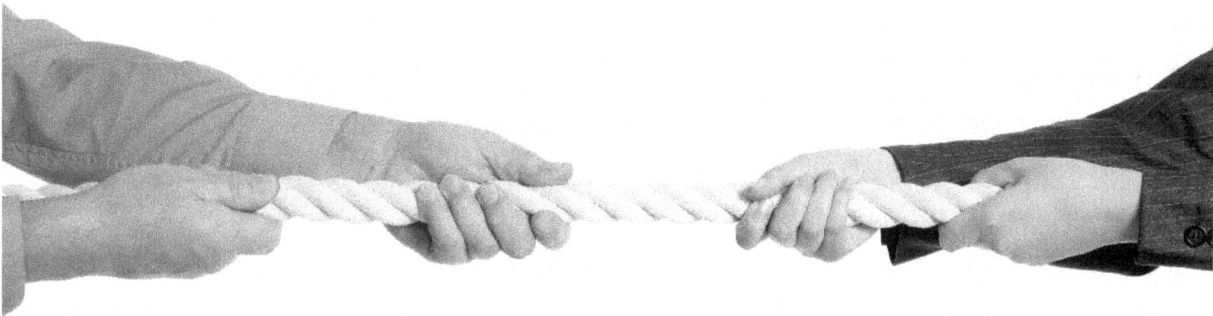

The struggle is real.

Weight loss is an arduous process.

Nonetheless, the concept is incredibly easy.

If you eat fewer calories than you burn, you are sure to lose weight.

Let's say you eat 1800 calories in your day. If you don't want to accumulate any fat from what you ate, you must do enough activities, exercises, movements, and efforts in your day to burn at least 1800 calories. If your daily energy consumption is of only 1500, then you will store 300 calories worth of fat. I know you don't want that!

So, eat the right quantities of nutritious food. Exercise sufficiently as to burn calories beyond what you consume, and you will be in business!

Don't be fooled by the diet pill companies that claim that you can lose 2-3 pounds per day, without even changing your eating habits.

You know deep down inside that it'll be a waste of your money because the pills will **never** work on their own.

Believing that you can eat in the same unhealthy way as you usually do, pop a few weight loss pills and expect to lose weight, is beyond irrational.

As a marketing tactic, the supplement companies will list **exotic**-sounding ingredients, and they will claim that they have fat burning properties.

Some might, in fact, have fat burning properties, but so does some natural foods.

What you need to remember is that they do not **magically** work on their own; you DO have to participate in the weight loss process.

Unfortunately, some women believe this hype because they want "easy" and taking a few pills a day is easy.

Cleaning up your diet and exercising takes some level of strength of character, and is most certainly more demanding than taking weight loss pills.

If you gained weight over a period of 3 years, or a few months, don't you find it logical that losing it will also take time?

Nobody wakes-up forty pounds heavier or lighter, those are 2 processes that take time.

Don't expect to lose twenty pounds in 3 days by following what is presented to you either; I do not make false promise.

Nonetheless, if you do what is suggested in this guide, you'll transform your body in 1 month.

Realize that in a perfect scenario, you might lose 3 to 4 pounds a week.

In 4 weeks, you'll lose about 8 pounds or maybe 12 if your metabolism is fast.

Believe me; you don't want to lose the weight too fast and end up with ugly flabby skin hanging under your arms, belly, and even your chin.

It all depends on your body. But strangely, the more excess weight you have, the faster you will lose weight. It's ironic, I know, but it is the way it usually goes.

Also, the leaner you will get, the more **challenging** it will become.

Whatever the case may be, 1 month is an appropriate time frame to aim for **noticeable** results.

Here is a fitness industry quote.

It takes 4 weeks for you to see your body changing.

It takes eight weeks for your friends and family to notice.

It takes twelve weeks for the rest of the world to see.

Keep going

In 1 month, the transformation that you will see will give you the motivation to keep going because you'll notice the difference and know that you are on the right path.

Most people expect instant results and give up when they don't get it.

Usually, they just haven't given themselves enough time.

You need to give yourself at least thirty days to see significant results.

You'll also need to plan your weight loss journey if you want to know how much time it will take you to reach your set goal.

We'll be looking at that in the next chapter.

What's important is that you keep things real for you.

Knowing that it will take you about eight weeks total to reach your ideal body weight, will motivate you to keep going, since, you'll know that if you're 2 weeks in, you'll only have 6 more weeks to go.

Nevertheless, you also will not believe the hype that the infomercials and supplements throw at you.

Your body works at its **own** pace. Everyone has a different metabolism.

It's not affected by hype or fantasies.

Weight loss is based on natural laws.

You **wear** what you **eat**. Think about that one.

Unquestionably, you need to move **more**, that might purely mean to dance a few times per week, go for walks, or run. What is more, you need to stay on course.

This is what **transforms** your body.

I know it doesn't seem very exciting or enjoyable, but believe me, this guide will show you ways to do all that in a fun and reasonable fashion... and you will lose weight.

In the following chapter, you'll learn how much time it'll take you to reach your desired weight.

Chapter 2

Plan and follow your progress

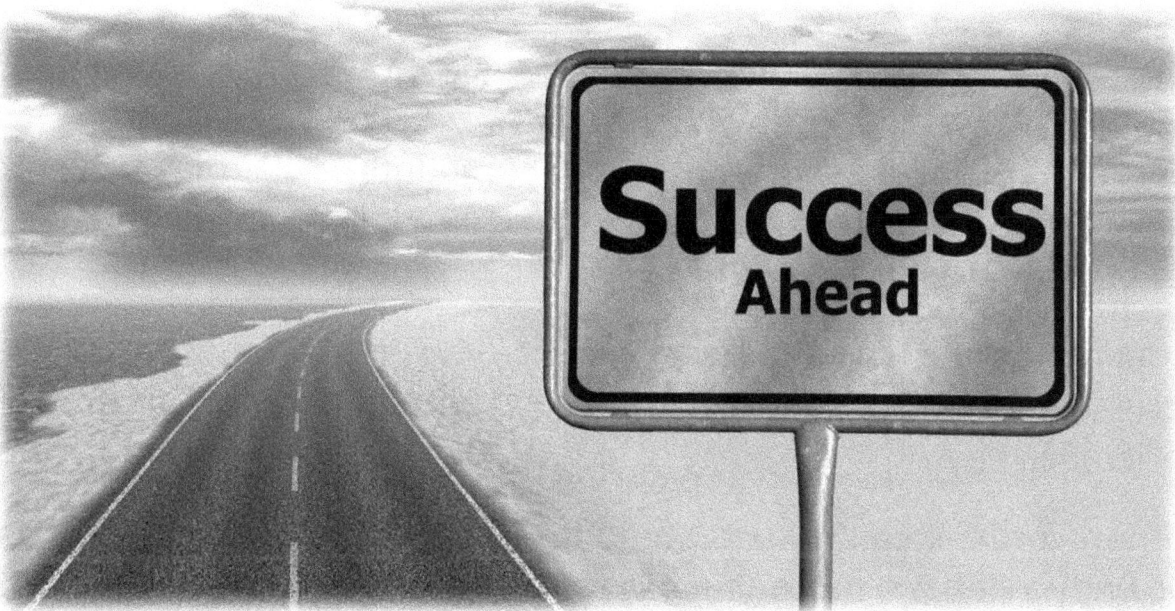

Enough preparation talk, now we'll get into the nitty-gritty.

Being aware of your daily caloric deficit is the first thing you should do.

You can go here and check that out.

http://www.freedieting.com/tools/calorie_calculator.htm

https://www.healthline.com/nutrition/how-many-calories-per-day

What truly matters most in a weight loss regiment is eating fewer calories than what it takes to maintain your present weight.

In other words, being at a daily caloric deficit is the essential factor that determines if you will **succeed** or fail.

You might eat super healthy with plenty of greens and salads and discover that you are not losing weight. That might be because you are eating more calories than is required for you to be at a weight loss caloric level.

This is the reason why so many people struggle to lose weight and never see progress. They are not eating in a caloric deficit manner.

What is a caloric deficit?

It merely means a shortage in the amount of calories consumed compared to the number of calories required for the maintenance of current body weight.

To maintain your current body weight, you might have to eat 1800 calories per day. But to lose weight, you will have to eat around 1300 calories per day.

In other words, if you're consuming fewer calories than your body uses, your body will have no choice but to tap into its fat supplies for fuel.

This is the only way you will diminish your body's stored fat and consequently lose weight.

Ideally, you should aim for a 500-calorie daily deficit.

You don't need to obsess over the numbers and aim for perfection.

If you're within the 400 to 600 range, you'll be perfectly fine, and you will lose weight **steadily**.

In order to **know** your daily caloric intake, you can visit this site.

http://www.freedieting.com/tools/calorie_calculator.htm

All you need to do is fill out the necessary fields and click on the "calculate" button.

You'll be shown 3 different numbers:

- **<u>Maintenance</u>** means that if you consume **this** number of calories, your weight will neither go up nor go down.

- **<u>Fat loss</u>** denotes a caloric **deficit. This is the number that you need to aim for in order to lose weight.**

- **<u>Extreme Fat Loss</u>** is an indicator that you should **not** drop your calories below this number.

Of course, if you eat more calories than the indicated maintenance level, you will inevitably gain weight.

Most quick fix weight loss method want you to aim for the extreme fat loss caloric intake. But that is too drastic. It is too much of a shock to your body.

It will result in flabby skin. Most of all, once you stop eating at a very low caloric intake, you will be at high risk of gaining back your weight faster than you lost it and then some.

How long will it take you to be at your desired weight?

If you wish to lose 20 pounds and you're losing about 2 pounds a week, which is, by the way, an excellent rate for constant weight loss, then you'll be looking at a time frame of 10 weeks, that is about 2 and a half months.

Does that seem too long for you?

Here's what **Earl Nightingale** once said – *"Don't let the fear of the time it will take to accomplish something, stand in the way of you doing it. The time will pass anyway; might as well put that passing time to the best possible use."*

Even if it takes you 10-15-20 weeks, as Nikes so eloquently says it "Just do it."

While this guide states that you will lose weight in 1 month, these 30 days are for **you** to see a transformation, not to reach your weight loss objective; unless you only need to lose 8 to 12 pounds.

Realize that most women **never** see any results.

...But if you follow this guide, YOU will see results.

However, if you need ten weeks to reach your goal, understand that you're not going to achieve it in 30 days. If we follow the example mentioned above, you'll lose 8 pounds in 1 month.

It may not seem like much, but it is definitely going to be a **visible** difference.

Your face will be slimmer. Your belly and thighs may seem like they have shrunk a little. You'll be amazed at the actual change. And you should feel immensely proud of yourself!

The whole point of this book is to show you what's possible and from there you just keep on going.

If it takes you 10-20-30 weeks, you keep doing what you've been doing these 30 days until you reach the desired goal.

One thing is sure; you must stay on track!

***

If you get the picture, you understand that you will have a better idea of how long it will take you to reach your set goal only once your first month is over.

Only then will you have the information you need to efficiently estimate the time it will take you to reach your anticipated weight.

Once you know how many pounds of fat you lose in a month, you will divide it by 4 and get your average weekly fat loss.

Take the amount of weight you want to lose and divide it by your weekly average.

Example: You want to lose 40 pounds. After your first month of healthy caloric deficit eating plus some physical activities, you lose 12 pounds per month, so that means 3 pounds per week.

40 divided by 3 = 13.33 weeks until you reach your goal. That is about 3 and a half months.

Isn't that amazing?!? Only 3 ½ months to lose 40 pounds!

Now I could make you believe that 1 pound of fat takes 4 times more space in your body than muscles, because if you Google it, you will find plenty of pictures showing you so.

But in truth, those pictures are comparing 5 pounds of fat with 1 pound of muscle. Remember that 1 pound is 1 pound.

In fact, fat is only 18% greater in volume, which is not that big of a difference visually. It IS more significant, but not as big as they make it out to be on those pictures plastered all over the web.

What I do want you to realize though is the equivalence of what your lost weight is compared to things you know.

1 pound	= a loaf of bread or a football
2 pounds	= 1 liter of milk or a pineapple
3 pounds	= a cardboard can of Crisco vegetable oil
5 pounds	= a bag of white sugar or a 2-liter bottle of soda
10 pounds	= a large bag of potatoes
15 pounds	= a 19" flat screen TV or a big bowling ball
20 pounds	= an automobile tire
25 pounds	= a container of cat litter
35 pounds	= the average car battery
40 pounds	= a 5-gallon bottle of water
50 pounds	= a small bale of hay
55 pounds	= a 5,000 BTU air conditioner
70 pounds	= a portable photo booth
85 pounds	= 17 watermelons
90 pounds	= 60 dozen eggs
95 pounds	= an average sized recliner chair
100 pounds	= a 2-month-old horse
150 pounds	= the complete Oxford English Dictionary
185 pounds	= Actor Hugh Jackman
200 pounds	= a typical refrigerator or a utility *hole cover*
250 pounds	= ten 25 pound bags of ice
300 pounds	= an average football lineman

Now, whatever weight you manage to lose, imagine holding the object that is equivalent to your lost weight. Realize that you use to carry that much weight around.

Another quirky fact, if you lose around 40 pounds or more, you might feel a slight pull from your belly-button. You may also notice that your organs are slightly sliding into its proper place.

That is an incredibly good sign.

Likewise, if you notice that you have not lost any weight on the scale for a while, but in the mirror, you unquestionably look slimmer, you are not hallucinating. Your body is going through some significant changes for the better. Once it has settled, you will start to see the pounds melting away again.

Tracking Your Progress

What gets quantified gets controlled.

Therefore, it's imperative that you measure your progress with **pictures, weighing scale, measuring tape, and tracking journal.**

This will ensure that you will keep a close eye on your diet and training.

The first thing you'll need to do is weigh yourself on a weighing scale. You should do this once a week on the **same day** and at the **same time**.

Do **not** weigh yourself daily because your weight **will** fluctuate, and it can be demoralizing. Once a week will do, and it will reflect any weight loss.

Do note that the scale weight only gives you a **general** idea, but it is not indicative of body composition.

For example, if you lost 3 pounds of fat and gained 2 pounds of muscle, the scale will only show a loss of 1 measly pound.

This can be very misleading. You'd actually have made excellent progress and will look different since fat does take up close to 20% more space than muscle.

That is why you also need to take **photos** of your body once every 2 weeks. With pictures, the difference in your appearance will be more evident, and you'll feel more motivated.

Many people are much more amazed to see before and after photos instead of just a difference in numbers on a scale.

Surprisingly, a woman's weight can actually fluctuate as much as 5 to 10 pounds overnight! Why is that, you may ask? Some of the reasons are because of the menstrual cycle, constipation, and water retention.

If you can ask your doctor to measure your body fat percentage by using calipers, you will then know by how much you will need to lower your body fat percentage to reach a level that is ideal for you.

No time to see your doctor? No worries.

You can use a soft measuring tape or what is called a seamstress measuring tape and gauge different parts of your body.

Put the tape around the middle of your thigh, and do the same for your arms, hips, chest, and even your neck.

To ensure accuracy, it's imperative that every time that you take down your measurements, it must be at the **same** place on your body.

Find specific markings on your body such as birthmarks, beauty marks, and use those as your guide to always measure at the same places. In your notebook, don't forget to write down what you used as your reference point. Example: Left thigh – where 3 beauty marks are forming a triangle.

Over time, you'll see the inches get smaller and smaller.

So even if after changing your eating habits and exercising for 2 weeks, the numbers on the scale are kind of discouraging, don't let that get to you because with the measuring tape, you'll get your proof that you did lose weight since the measurement will shrink down.

Remember, muscles are 18% denser than fat, and they also don't occupy as much space.

Be aware that the results are usually slower in the first 3-4 weeks. You'll probably feel like you are doing something wrong, and you might want to give up right then and there, but don't!

Changes are happening within you.

Your metabolic rate is increasing, and your body is adapting to your new way of life. It is starting to use its stored fat as energy.

On the inside, a lot of things are happening even though you cannot see visible results on the outside; **yet**.

This discourages many women who quit their weight loss program within the first month. In fact, most give up after 2 weeks!

They take a break and go back to their poor eating habits and sedentary lifestyle. 2 months later, they decide to give it another try to lose weight again.

When does it ever end?

This is the biggest mistake a dieter can do. As the pedal hits the metal and results are about to show, you stop everything!

Remember; Your motivation gives you the fuel to start, then habit kicks in and your good to go all the way to your goal.

When you finally decide to venture on a health and weight loss journey, you should fix a retrospect date. You could choose to make your review date 90 days later. Once you've decided for a review time, continue until you've completed it or in this example don't stop until you've reached your 3 month period or until you are at your intended weight; whichever comes first.

Realize that there may be occasions where you will slip-up on your diet. There may be times when you won't have time to workout. There may even be weeks where there will be no change in weight.

Despite all these, keep going until you reach the 90-day mark.

Then, according to your results, you can adjust and decide to go on for another set time.

If you've reached your goal, congratulations!!! Now your new goal is to maintain that weight by eating at a maintenance level and continue with some physical activities to stay healthy and to burn calories.

If you think you're done, that's it, that's all, you will soon see your weight start to creep back on. You should see weight loss as a series of small goals that you achieve one after the other.

One thing is for sure; if you hate starting over, stop giving up.

In 3 short months, you will be so glad you stuck to it.

So don't surrender and kill off your excellent health and weight loss dreams before they have time to bloom.

Every week, track your progress, and if you are not losing weight, adjust your diet and your workout plan.

Exercise a little bit more and slightly reduce your calorie intake.

This is the best way to lose weight without losing your way.

Chapter 3

Curbing your appetite holistically

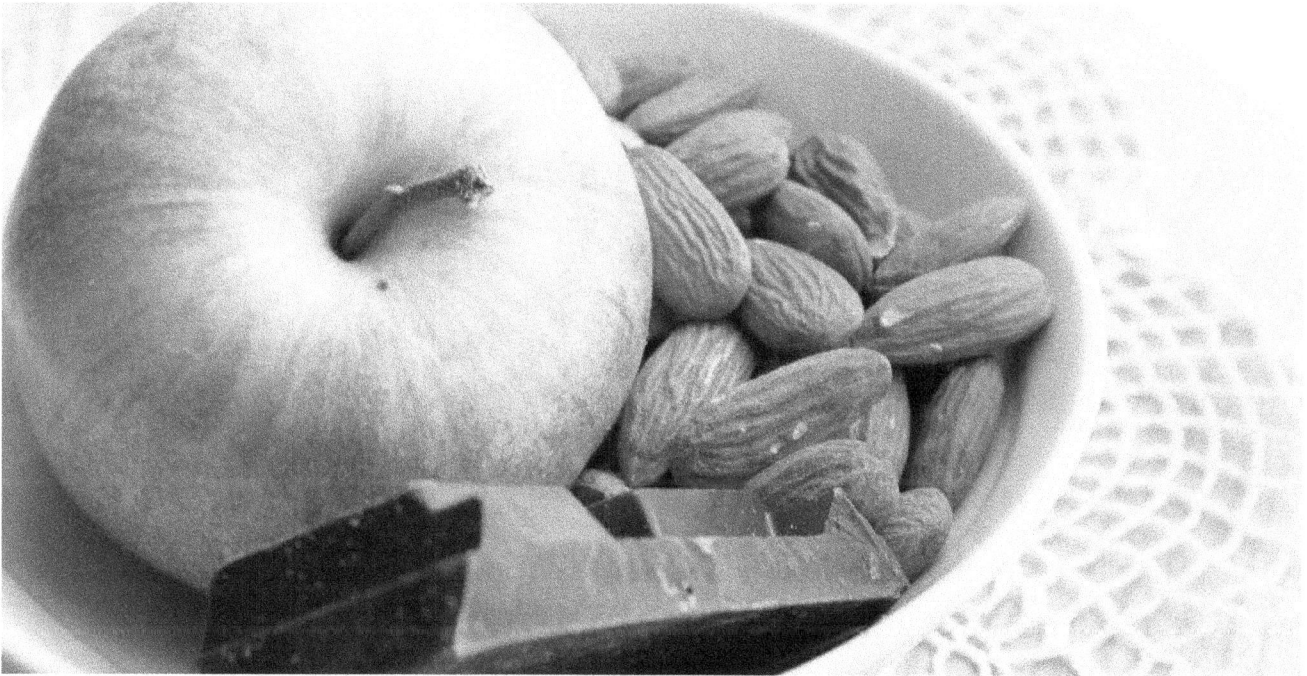

You cannot avoid it. To lose weight, you must reduce your food intake or opt for low-calorie food that you can eat in significant quantities.

I know you don't want to eat less. You enjoy eating too much.

- Do I really have to cut down my calorie intake?

Yes. You really, really do.

- What if I eat the same amount of food and exercise?

No. You still need to eat less.

- Ok, ok. Let's say, I eat the same amount, exercise like crazy and pop a few slimming pills as well. That's ok? Right?

No. You'll still have to eat less.

Hoping that the facts are now well established, we can continue to more stimulating subjects.

When we say you have to eat less, it doesn't mean that you'll have to starve yourself

You'll always eat enough to feel satiated, stay strong, and healthy.

Society's problem these days is that people overeat.

People eat when they're happy. People eat when they're depressed.

They eat when they're hungry, and they also eat when they're NOT hungry... out of fear that they might get hungry later.

I know you've been there.

Once you aim to cut your calories, you will most certainly eat less than you usually do. Because you're in the habit of consuming a certain quantity of food daily, the body is, of course, going to feel a little hungry.

This is a normal feeling. You're not starving. Your body simply requires time to adjust to the fewer calories it is ingesting. You will probably feel some discomfort in the first few days, and you may find yourself thinking of food, **often**. Therefore, you will need to exercise **will-power** and not eat.

Maintaining a caloric deficit is imperative to losing the pounds.

There are **eight tips** in this chapter to help you reduce your calorie intake and curb your appetite. These are **crucial** pointers that are the back-bones of your "diet."

They will facilitate, to a certain extent, by controlling your cravings.

Don't worry, after a week of cutting down your calories, your stomach will seem to have shrunken and your appetite will lessen.

It is true what people say that the less you eat, the less you need or want to eat. You will feel full with much less food.

Now, that is fantastic news, don't you think?

Give it a week or 2, max, and things will fall into place. Of course, the more you are used to eating a lot, the longer it will take, but the further along you are in your journey to health, the less food you'll need.

7 Tips to Curbing Hunger

Skip breakfast.

I know, I know, this runs contrary to everything you've heard for the past few decades. But you see, some studies have demonstrated that if you eat your first meal as late as possible, the less you'll eat that day. Makes sense, since you end up not eating those morning calories. If skipping breakfast is too tricky for you, go ahead and have a light breakfast, but don't forget to make it protein base, so that you can feel satiated longer. By all means, avoid sugary cereals and any bread.

Drink lots of water.

By drinking a lot of water, you will feel full. Often thirst is disguised as hunger. Besides, to accelerate fat loss, being well hydrated is a must.

Keep moving all day

Watching TV for hours on end and playing video games does not help you burn off the calories you consume. Also, those are activities that make you want to munch constantly. Avoid them as much as possible, unless you are paying some sort of physical video game like a type of dance off.

Eat heaps of vegetables.

Vegetables such as **broccoli, spinach, carrots, cauliflower, kale, celery,** etc. contain a ton of beneficial properties. Not only are they good for your health, but they will also leave you feeling **fuller for longer** because of all the fiber that they contain. Eating them raw, is even better!

Small plates are the key

This is mostly psychological, as the smaller your plate is, the fuller it'll look. That sends a signal to your brain that you are eating a full plate. Hence you are eating a lot, but that is not the case, so you'll eat fewer calories.

Take your time.

Countless times over the last decades, it has been proven that it takes about 20 minutes before the brain can detect that the stomach is full. So, one way of not overeating is to take your time. Savor your food.

Early to bed

Chances are quite high that if you are not in bed by 9 pm, you will want to pop some junk food in your mouth. Why? You say. Because you'll most likely be watching TV or a movie, and 99% of the time it'll mean that you will want to snack on something while doing that. Go to bed early; avoid useless calories.

Follow the tips above, and you will **reduce** the amount of food that you eat.

Once you achieve this feat, your weight loss will go from being a possibility to a reality.

Your diminished food intake is "that" essential to your success.

Never forget that.

Take the time to plan to exercise, plan to prepare healthy meals, plan to drink your water, and plan to go to bed on time.

Planning keeps us inline. If you don't plan, you will be inconsistent, all over the place, and might fall off track.

Likewise, anyone who wants to lose 50lb or more needs to approach losing weight more holistically.

Doesn't that sound exotic and mysterious?

It merely means that you must see your weight loss as a whole.

You must decide to make changes across many areas of your life.

It's not JUST about exercise and eating right. It takes a step by step approach that is complete, rounded.

Therefore, you must have the right attitude, meditate, plan your meals, exercise, and surround yourself with healthy people that are in great shape.

That is what I mean by a rounded approach. It covers all the bases, and it is done incrementally.

If you drastically stop eating all that you are used to, if you exercise like crazy, if you give up all your juice and soft drinks at once, you will quickly fizzle out and give up.

Doing it incrementally is the key.

To help you figure out the calories that you eat, here is a practical food calorie calculator.

https://www.webmd.com/diet/healthtool-food-calorie-counter

Sometimes it is just easier to google what you eat to get the number of calories in the item. Example: calories in 2 cups of pasta

The link below is also an excellent place to get the calorie count in food.

https://www.nutritionix.com/

Food diary template

https://www.vertex42.com/ExcelTemplates/food-diary-template.html

When you first start out filling your food diary, you might find it time-consuming to calculate all the calories that you eat. But after a week or 2 of eating your favorite healthy foods, you won't have to calculate anymore.

You will already know the calorie counts of most meals and snacks that you consume.

Let's say that most mornings you have a bowl of oatmeal, it then becomes quick and easy to fill in the calorie info in your journal.

Chapter 4

Fat burning food

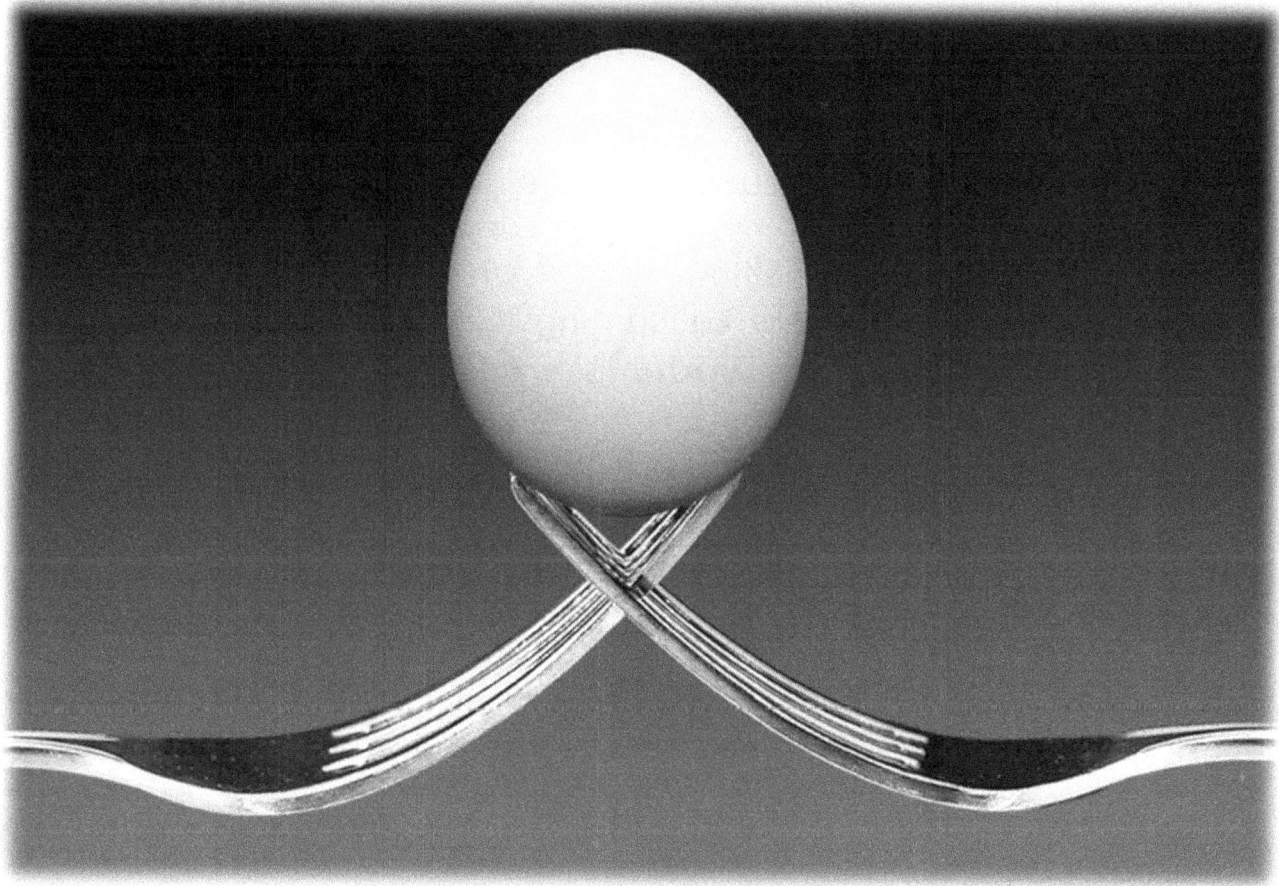

You don't need to diet, but you do need to **change** your diet.

I know that sound quite baffling.

Many women make the mistake of starving themselves in the hope of losing weight fast. This is **counterproductive** and works against them.

You need to be on a particular food intake regiment that is right for **you**, and most importantly, you need to be at a **caloric deficit**.

As long as you're at a caloric deficit, you **will** lose weight.

Did I say it enough times yet?

You're probably wondering, ***"What if I ate junk food and still maintained a caloric deficit?"***

In theory, yes, you would lose weight. It's not that simple, but yes. You can lose weight even while eating fast food, processed food, or junk food, whatever you may call it. You know what these foods are.

As was mentioned in chapter 1, if you consume lesser calories than your **maintenance** level, you will lose weight.

Therefore, theoretically speaking, even if you were on a junk food diet the entire day, but you were consuming about 500 calories less than your maintenance level, you **would** lose weight.

Many overweight or obese women frequently have an extremely poor diet. It is particularly challenging for them to switch from a menu that is so high in processed and junk food, to one that is clean and wholesome.

Expecting to switch your diet overnight is just setting yourself up for failure. You absolutely must do this **slowly** and progressively.

Therefore, your best course of action will be to carry on eating the way you have but aim for a caloric deficit.

That essentially means that you'll be consuming less junk food than you were used to. This, in itself, will help you lose weight.

However, since the goal is to lose weight AND get healthy, your end goal should be to eliminate junk food from your diet and eat clean.

That being said, every week, you should make 1 or 2 small positive changes to the way you eat.

Don't diet; change your habits

If you usually have 2 cheeseburgers for lunch followed by a soda, you may replace those cheeseburgers with a lean chicken or crunchy tuna wrap and a glass of water or green tea.

Psychologically, this is easier. It's just 1 meal. Keep at it until this becomes a habit and you slowly but surely, replace all the junk meals with wholesome yet tasty meals.

Healthy meals can be delicious too. You are not sacrificing taste or pleasure by eating nutritiously. It's just a matter of getting your taste buds and body to enjoy eating healthy foods. Over time this will be achieved.

Meanwhile, if you decide to only eat junk food but you maintain a caloric deficit, you will lose some weight.

But remember one thing, junk food lacks nutrients.

Which means, a short while after eating junk food, you will feel hungry again.

That's because your body needs certain nutrients to strive, and if it doesn't get it, it screams hunger!

It will happen every time you eat a poor diet; you will constantly feel hungry. Thus, you will eat more and gain weight.

Also, note that specific processes within the body will prevent you from losing weight beyond a certain point.

The body is an extraordinarily intricate system. Since you are following a caloric deficit diet, it WILL lose weight for a certain period. However, don't fool yourself, thinking it will continue as such. Over time it will be harder and harder to lose an ounce.

Losing weight is not a simple mathematical equation. Even if you do eat at a caloric deficit, other factors are involved, such as the quality of the calories eaten. The thermogenic effect of certain food is also a big factor.

So, if you are a junk food enthusiast, you should ideally continue eating what you like, at a caloric deficit of course, and over the course of a month or 2, slowly transition to healthier foods until your diet is filled with healthy, nutrient-rich food.

Once in a while, you may, of course, treat yourself to not so healthy cuisine, such as cake, pizza, fries, etc. But you will find that over time you won't even feel the urge to eat junk food. Believe me, that day is not so far away if you start today and keep an open mind.

One of the best ways of eating to lose weight will be to consume foods that help with the **fat burning process**.

By including these foods in your diet, you'll not only feel more satiated, but the body will burn more calories too. Unlike weight loss supplements, these foods actually work… and they're much cheaper.

Foods that burn fat

- Almonds

- Oatmeal

- Eggs

- Legumes & Beans

- Berries

- Olive oil

- Coconut oil

- Green vegetables

- Lean meats & oily fish

- Green tea

- Avocados

- All-natural peanut butter

By consuming the foods mentioned above, you'll naturally curb your hunger, and you'll also hasten the fat burning process.

So… while you do not need to follow a highly restricted diet and starve yourself, you should aim to consume foods that are **beneficial** to your health.

You won't believe how much food you'll be able to eat if it's natural and unprocessed.

Chapter 5

Holding back the Carbs

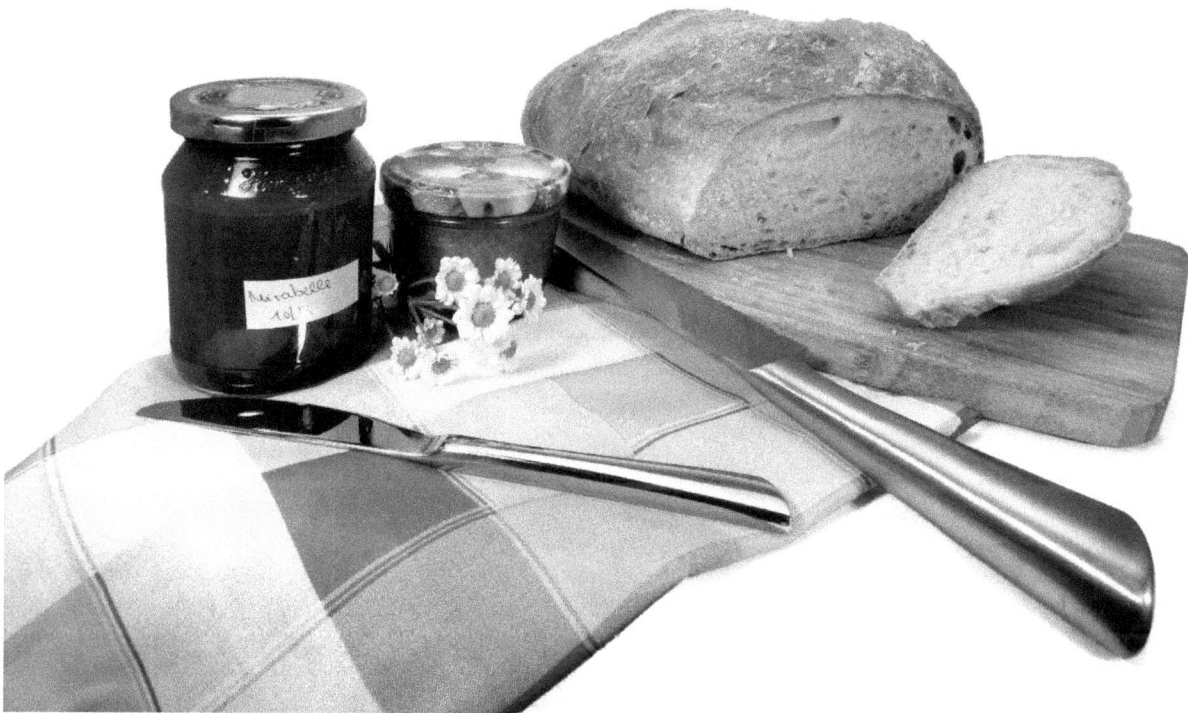

Before telling you what are the right foods to eat, here is 1 of the BEST ways to lose weight fast.

This is a major one!

Cut Your Intake of Carbs

Carbohydrate intake is one of the **most significant** factors affecting the **speed** at which you lose weight. In fact, the main reason most women gain weight is that they consume **too much processed carbs.**

When you eat processed carbs such as **donuts, pasta, white bread,** etc. the calories quickly add up, and the body has too much fuel.

The body shuttles all the excess fuel, produced by eating too many carbs, into its fat stores. That's how you gain weight.

Furthermore, processed carbs usually cause a spike in insulin levels, which indirectly lead to **weight gain**.

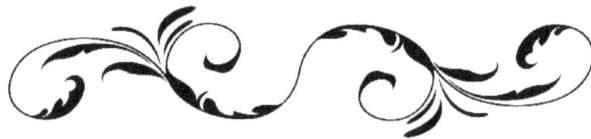

As mentioned before, one of the best ways to lose some fat is without a doubt, by restricting your carb intake. As a matter of fact, studies have shown that diminishing one's carb intake is even more efficient than restricting calories.

Did I really say that? I sure did!

So, if you're on a 500-calorie daily deficit, and your carb intake is also minimal, you have a lot more chances of losing twice the weight in the same period than you would by consuming carbs while on a caloric deficit diet alone.

Now, you may be thinking, "That is all fine and dandy" ...

- But what exactly ARE carbs anyway???

Glad you asked!

Carbohydrates are essential nutrients found in numerous types of foods.

Most of us equate carbs with bread and pasta, but you can also find them in:

- dairy products
- sweets, snack foods, sodas, juice drinks, cakes, cookies, candy, chips
- fruits and juices
- starchy vegetables like potatoes, peas, and corn
- grains like rice, oatmeal, and barley
- nuts
- legumes, dried beans like pinto beans and soy products like veggie burgers
- seeds
- grain-based foods like bread, cereal, pasta, and crackers
- and so many more.

Non-starchy vegetables like lettuce, cucumbers, broccoli, and cauliflower have **minimal** carbohydrates and minimal impact on your blood glucose. Those are what we call **good carbs**.

Consuming healthy carbs is very beneficiary for our body. Glucose (a form of sugar) produced by the consumption of carbs moves in around the body through your bloodstream and is the main source of food for the brain, muscles, and other vital cells.

3 components make up carbohydrates: fiber, starch, and sugar.

Complex carbs, in other words, good carbs, are made of fiber and starch. As for the bad carbs, they are merely sugar.

The body can process simple carbs very fast since it consists of simple molecular structures. It's easily and very quickly digested, so you get a boost of energy, but it doesn't last, which mean you get hungry again, thus eat more, it's a vicious cycle.

Added sugar, such as the kind that you add to your food, offer no nutritional value. They are empty calories. Simply put, you eat something that offers no beneficial vitamins, fibers, or minerals. You are eating food that will only cause fat to accumulate in our body.

Simple Carbohydrates vs. Complex Carbohydrates

You may have heard that eating **complex carbs** is better than **simple carbs**, which is true since foods containing complex carbohydrates are processed more slowly by the body and provide sustained energy levels over more extended periods of time.

Foods rich in healthy **complex carbohydrates** include

- Whole grains
- Wholemeal bread
- Wholegrain breakfast cereals
- Oats
- Wholegrain pasta
- Brown rice
- Potatoes
- Beans
- Lentils
- Chickpeas

To get back to the point, when you cut down your carb intake, your body will burn more fat from its **fat supplies** because it doesn't have many carbs to burn as fuel.

That is great news because it means that your body will burn fat much faster.

Your body's blood sugar level will drop, and people who have diabetes will see an improvement in their condition. A restrictive carb diet also keeps type 2 diabetes at bay since the body's insulin sensitivity is sound.

Your good cholesterol levels will also go up, and your bad cholesterol levels will drop.

Many people assume that cholesterol is linked to fat intake.

The truth is that a high carb intake also harms your cholesterol levels. This runs contrary to widespread belief, yet studies show that a **low-carb** diet has more positive effects on your triglycerides than a **low-fat** diet.

When you think of fat developing and being stored in your hips or stomach, you're thinking of triglycerides.

Any calories your body doesn't need to use right away is converted into triglycerides. The triglycerides are warehoused in your fat cells.

Later, hormones caused by real hunger, or by exercising, release triglycerides for energy between meals, making you lose some weight.

That being said, it is essential to note that **you should never take things to extremes**. This applies to carb restriction as well.

Certain diets, such as the Atkins diet, restrict the consumption of carbs for a long period. That is harmful to your body. You will feel tremendous fatigue on top of being moody and weak.

Such a diet is not sustainable, and once you stop that type of diet, you will gain whatever weight you lost and more.

An excessive restriction of carbs for a prolonged period, will not only compromise your immune system, but it will also lead to muscle loss, it will slow down your fat burning process and worst of all, it will put you on a weight loss plateau. Nobody wants to be stuck there.

If that wasn't enough, your body will dramatically reduce its testosterone production, even if you are a woman, and this is lethal for your thyroid,. What's more, you will develop a leptin resistance, which will lead you to gain weight once more. We will talk more about leptin resistance later on in this guide.

So, what can you do? How are you supposed to hit the right balance?

You want the best of both worlds, don't you?

The only way to achieve this is with a technique that is known as **carb cycling**.

How to do Carb cycling?

You will avoid carbohydrates for **3 to 6 days** at a time.

If you have more then 50 pounds to lose, you probably have a slower metabolism then most. You should aim for 5 to 6 days of minimal or zero carbs.

You will get a much faster result eating only around 50 to 150 grams of carbs per day, not more.

If you only have a few extra pounds to lose, you need to go for 3 to 4 days with low or no carbs.

After the period of carb restriction is over, you will follow it with 1 day of carb intake. This is known as your "**re-feed**" or "**re-fuel**" day.

Consume reasonable amounts of carbs on that day to give your body the fuel that it needs.

Your metabolism will get a **boost** and your body will get a surge of energy as its fuel stores get replenished.

How much is a reasonable amount of carb?

In Re-fuel mode, you should aim to eat between 225 to 325 grams of carbs and **500 to 700 calorie surplus <u>over maintenance level</u>**.

This will put your body back into fat burning mode.

Stick to healthy carbs such as:

• Oatmeal (old-fashioned or Steel Cut)	100g=12g of carbs
• Yams (similar to sweet potatoes)	100g=28g of carbs
• Brown rice	100g=23g of carbs
• Sweet potatoes	100g=20g of carbs
• Multigrain hot cereal	100g=38g of carbs
• White potatoes with skin	1 large=64g of carbs
• 100% whole wheat bread	100g=41g of carbs
• 100% whole wheat pasta	250g cook=37g of carbs
• Beans and lentils	100g=20g of carbs
• Cream of rice hot cereal	100g=11g of carbs
• Quinoa	1 cup=39g of carbs
• Couscous	100g=23g of carbs
• Pumpkin	100g=7g of carbs
• Butternut squash	100g=12g of carbs
• Fresh Beets	100g=10g of carbs
• Bananas	100g=23g of carbs
• Oranges	100g=12g of carbs
• Blueberries	100g=14g of carbs
• Grapefruits	100g=11g of carbs
• Apples	100g=14g of carbs

To accelerate your fat loss, use this technique repeatedly. You will improve your health, and come down of your weight loss plateau.

For that purpose, here are a few carb counters to help you gage your intake of carbs.

http://www.carb-counter.org/veg/

https://ketologic.com/carbcounter/

https://www.carb-counter.net/

With this method, there will come a day when you won't even crave for carbs or junk food anymore. Won't that be great!

Your tastes in food will change the more your body gets healthy. That's why fit people are consistently able to make wise food choices. Once you have gotten over the hump of ditching these addictive foods, the rest is easy.

Your insulin sensitivity will improve, the pounds will drop, and you will **look and feel** like a brand new you.

Chapter 6

Pay attention to what you eat

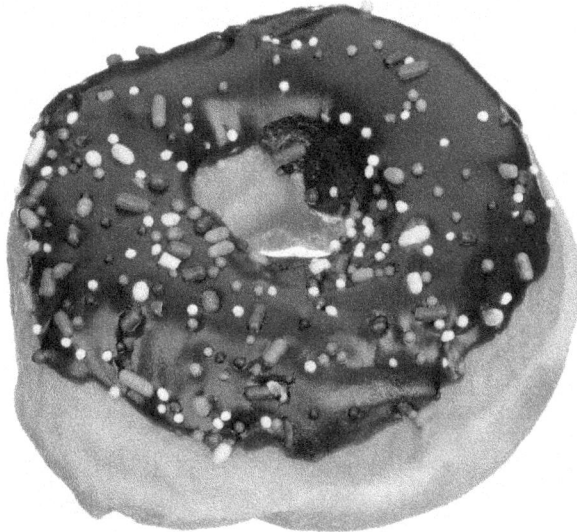

When it comes to weight loss, most of your focus must be given to what you eat.

The 7 foods listed below will literally sabotage your weight loss efforts.

There is absolutely no doubt that you have everything to gain and nothing to lose, but fat, by avoiding these foods.

The glitch in that instance is that many people love these comfort foods way too much to give them up.

Sugar is addictive.

The more sugary foods you eat, the more you'll crave it.

However, by eliminating them **slowly**, you'll gradually condition your body to crave for healthier food.

7 Foods you should avoid at all costs!

- **Doughnuts:** Consisting of nothing more than refined carbohydrates and sugar, they are probably 1 of the unhealthiest foods on the planet.

  They are high in calories, fats, carbs, and other preservatives. Long term ingestion of doughnuts is a sure way to gain weight and to suffer from digestion problems.

- **Fast food:** They lack in nutrition; they make you fat and are addictive.

- **Chips:** Who doesn't like chips? Not many people. After eating just 1 of those crunchy, salty pleasures, most people cannot stop themselves from eating way more then they should.

  But chips have high levels of trans fats, that is because of the hydrogenated vegetable oils used to fry them. This leads to cardiovascular disease and, you guessed it, weight gain.

- **French fries:** High in trans fats and carcinogens; besides making you gain weight, these foods can cause cancer.

- **Bagels:** Here is another crowd pleaser. It has an extremely high glycemic index. It causes insulin spikes, which creates inflammation in the body, along with other health issues like acne, body aches, clogged arteries, mood swings, etc. Those are all side effects of unstable insulin levels... and of course, it causes weight gain.

- **Microwaved popcorn:** A favorite amongst movies lovers. Convenient, tasty, and fun. Yet, they contain carcinogens and diacetyl — both which cause cancer.

- **Cereals:** A fat gaining culprit. Most cereals are not suitable for your body despite being marketed as "healthy natural foods."

   There is hardly anything natural about cereals. They are made with genetically modified grains that can harm you in the long run.

Just avoiding these unhealthy foods is half the battle won.

Always remember the long-term effects.

Don't give in to **sinful pleasures** in the short term, which may eventually lead to suffering.

Chapter 7

Power packed proteins

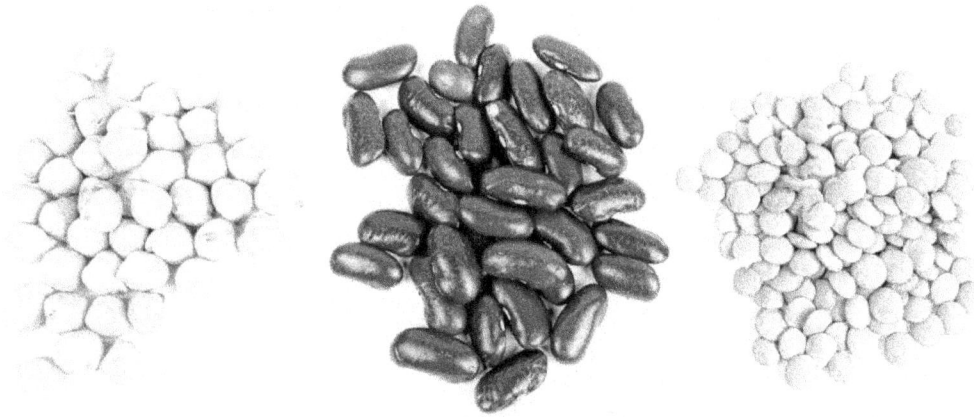

The following is one of the most powerful techniques to speed up weight loss.

The more proteins you consume, the faster you'll lose weight.

It takes much longer to digest protein, which in turn makes you feel full longer, and compared to simple carbs, the body burns a lot more calories just digesting it.

That entails that you should be getting quite a bit of your daily calories from **protein foods.**

Meats and legumes are fantastic sources of protein.

The protein will also help you gain muscle if you are on a weight training program. Aim for about 0.8 grams of protein per pound of body weight per day.

The protein will help build more muscle, and the great thing about that is that the more you have muscles, the more you will burn fat automatically.

It'll be like being on a fat burning auto-pilot.

This is an excellent cycle to be in. That is why you may notice that people who are muscular and fit get away with <u>eating more</u>.

Their muscles are **burning** more calories around the clock.

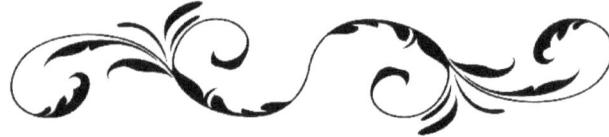

Seriously remember the following

- **Never consume a carb without a protein**.
  o For example: no pasta or bread without meat or beans
- **Never consume a fat without a protein.**
  o For example: no fatty meat or butter without beans, or cottage cheese

By simply having the protein together with these foods, you'll prevent an insulin spike.

Do you know what is one of the best ways to get protein in your diet?

The answer is inside the shell.

Eggs are 1 of the most nutritious foods on the planet. In the past, they have received a bad rap about high cholesterol and a lot of other false information.

This is highly ironic since cereals, which are detrimental to one's health, are believed to be healthy, while eggs, which are hugely beneficial, are demonized.

Let's set the record straight. Eggs are an excellent source of protein, omega-3 fatty acids and a lot of other beneficial nutrients.

Dietary cholesterol does not produce cholesterol in the body. Saturated fats and trans fat are the true culprits.

What this means is that eating whole eggs is perfectly fine. The yolk is not your enemy; on the contrary, all the nutrients of eggs are mostly found in the yolk.

In fact, eggs are considered by many nutritionists to be the **perfect food**.

Besides being a remarkable source of lean protein and omega-3 fatty acids, it also contains vitamin D, B6, B12, Choline, leucine, L-argi9, and folate.

You may not be familiar with what most of these vitamins are but what really matters is that they are what your body truly needs.

What really **does** matter is how the eggs are prepared and that you don't go overboard in consuming them.

So please don't fry your eggs in saturated fat or vegetable oils. Use coconut oil or olive oil. Fry them lightly or half-boil them.

Though egg yolks are high in protein, they are also calorie dense. So, if you want the benefit that eggs provide, but you do not want to add too many calories to your diet, don't eat more than 2 egg yolks in 1 meal.

One interesting point to note is that if you are consuming eggs everyday, your protein intake will be met and then some.

So, that being said, avoiding protein shakes and other commercially sold protein products, even those sold in health stores would be best if you are consuming eggs or high protein food.

If you can get your protein from a natural source, such as eggs, that is always ideal. Also, if you can, try to get organic eggs since they will contain less omega-6 fats and more of the incredibly good for the brain omega-3 fats.

If you're Vegan, many vegetables are high in protein as well.

By opting for high protein content veggies and legumes, you will meet the daily recommended intake.

20 Veggies high in protein

Edamame	18 g per cup
Lentils	18 g per cup
Lima Beans (Cooked)	11.6 g per cup
Soy sprout	9.2 g per cup
Peas (Green)	8.5 g per cup
Sprouted Beans	6 g per cup
Spinach (Cooked)	5.3 g per cup
Snap peas (cooked)	5.2 g per cup
Potato (with skin)	5 g per 1 medium potato
Sweet Corn (Yellow)	4.68 g per cup
Asparagus (cooked)	4.3g per cup
Artichokes	4.2g
Brussels Sprouts (Cooked)	4 g per cup
Broccoli	4 g per stalk (medium)
Kale (cooked)	3 g per cup
Mushrooms (White, cooked)	3 g per cup
Avocado (medium)	2.67g

When the goal is to transition to healthier foods, then whole foods must be the prevalent choice instead of the chemically filled processed foods.

A trick to remember is that generally speaking, whole foods are found on the perimeter of most supermarkets.

If you **avoid** the food in the inner aisles and shelves, you'll be distancing yourself away from the processed foods.

***

Remember that the 2 critical components to any fat loss regiment are being on a **caloric deficit** while on a balanced diet and adding a simple **exercise program**.

Everything else is just the icing on the cake.

So, no matter how healthy and clean your diet is, make sure you're still at a <u>daily caloric deficit.</u>

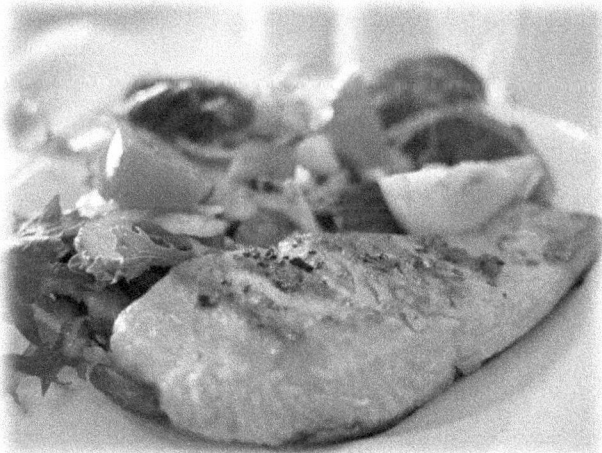

Good sources of protein

3 oz Chicken breast, no skin	24 g protein 284 calories
3 oz cooked beef 10% fat	22 g protein 184 calories
3 oz Salmon	19 g protein 175 calories
½ cup raw Oats	13 g protein 303 calories
1 cup Chickpeas	39 g protein 729 calories
1 oz can Sardines	7 g protein 59 calories
1 oz Tuna (154 g)	5.5 g protein 24 calories
1 large egg	6 g protein 78 calories

Fish contains Omega-3 fatty acids. That makes them even more beneficial to the body. They are particularly favorable in preventing and managing heart diseases.

Foods that trigger fat loss

The natural properties in certain foods trigger off specific processes in the body that literally cause fat loss. With this in mind, eating these foods will make your body **wake up** and <u>burn more fat.</u>

Here are but a few.

- Fatty fish

- MCT oils (look it up)

- Coffee

- Eggs

- Olive oil and Coconut oil

- Whey protein

- Apple cider vinegar

- Chili peppers

- Oolong tea and Matcha

- Full-fat Greek yogurt

Here are a few food items containing powerful antioxidants and nutrients which strengthen the immune system. To workout efficiently and burn more fat, you need to be well supported by a full range of nourishing food.

Other beneficial foods

- Red bell peppers are packed with vitamin c, almost twice as much as citrus

- All citrus fruits such as lemons, oranges, grapefruits, are bursting with vitamin C which help fight infection

- Broccoli is crammed with vitamins A, C, and E, and many other antioxidants and fiber. Broccoli is 1 of the healthiest vegetables you can eat.

- Turmeric (curcumin) rich in antioxidants and has strong anti-inflammatory properties

- Garlic and onions may help lower blood pressure and slow down hardening of the arteries

- Ginger may help decrease inflammation

- Spinach is filled with vitamin C, antioxidants, and beta carotene, which may increase the infection-fighting abilities of your body.

- Green tea packed with flavonoids and EGCG, which enhances immune function

When embarking on a weight loss journey, many women struggle with hunger.

You may find that those first 2 weeks are the hardest.

Always thinking of food can take a toll on your concentration and your willpower.

One of the ways you can prevent this undesirable feeling is by consuming foods that are high in fiber and therefore digest more slowly.

You will feel full for a longer period of time. Therefore, you will consume fewer calories without feeling hunger.

Foods high in fiber

• Oatmeal	• Pears
• Oats	• Apples
• Chia	• Prunes
• Buckwheat	• Oranges
• Quinoa	• Bananas
• Almonds	• Bran-flakes
• Beans	• Pearled Barley
• Lentils	• Whole wheat pasta
• Brown rice	• Artichokes
• Whole grain bread	• Potatoes
• Raspberries	• Spinach
• Avocados	• Carrots
• Broccoli	• Brussels sprouts

Chapter 8

Benefits of ON & OFF fasting

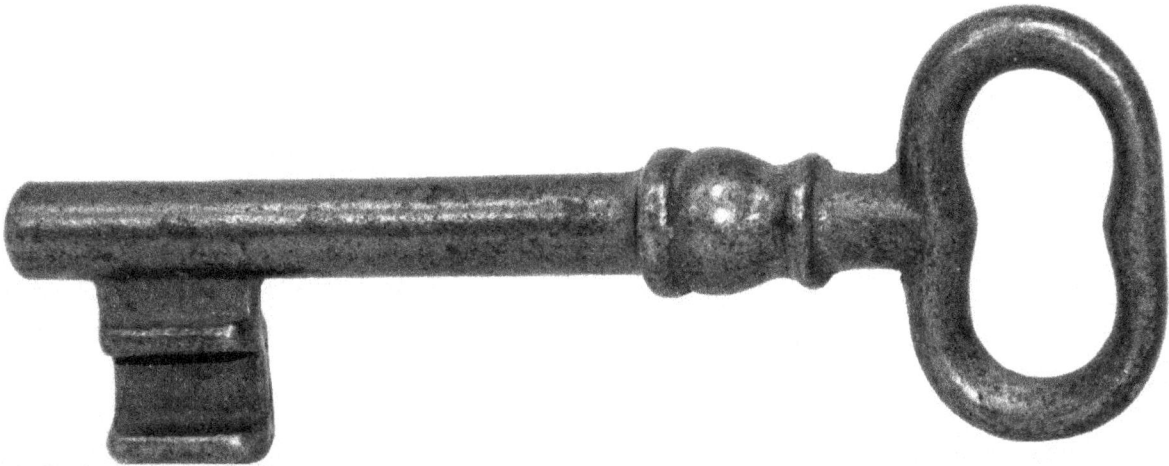

Even though Intermittent Fasting has been around for centuries, it is still 1 of the most scientifically proven successful ways of losing weight.

Defined by refraining from eating for specific fixed periods, it is the simplest way to boost your metabolism and lose weight.

A few of the physical benefits of fasting

- Improved mental clarity and concentration
- Fat loss
- Lowered blood insulin and sugar levels
- Reversal of type 2 diabetes
- Increased energy
- Increased growth hormone
- Lowered blood cholesterol
- Reduction of inflammation, thus reducing pain
- Reduction of seizures

Intermittent fasting is so effective and powerful that it may even help in Cancer prevention and treatment.

Exercise and fasting release the neurotransmitter norepinephrine from nerve terminals in the fat tissue; thereby stimulating triglyceride release.

In layman's terms, exercises, and fasting triggers the particular hormone that makes your fat cells release their fat. Thus, helping you lose weight.

Hormonal triggers that make the difference between gaining weight or burning fat are produced by the pancreas, which secretes 2 hormones called insulin and glucagon.

The combination of increased glucagon and decreased insulin levels in the blood caused by fasting is the hormonal signal that triggers the **release of fat cells**.

You may be thinking that this is way to easy to be effective, or you may also think that this sounds totally and outrageously absurd.

The only way to convince you of the magic of intermittent fasting is simply by trying it yourself.

This is the solution to when you feel that you've hit a weight loss plateau or when you slip-up and want to get back on track. Personally, I love to do intermittent fasting the day after I've indulged myself, or after a night on the town.

In fact, On & Off fasting allows you to eat more of what you love followed by a short fast.

One of the most popular fasting windows is simply to stop eating after 7 pm and not eat again until the next day between 5 and 7 pm. Or, simply skip breakfast for 2 days in a row.
The longer you fast, the more it gives your body the rest it needs and the ability to regenerate and replenish itself smoothly.

It allows faster weight loss, increases energy, can help reverse type 2 diabetes and many other benefits.

On top of all that you'll save time and money by doing On & Off fasting; Time, because you don't have to cook and money because you don't have to buy food or anything special to do it.

Fasting doesn't mean starving. Starving is when you have no other choice but not to eat, you don't control it. You have no food supplies. You lack nutrients, vitamins and so on... you therefor are starving.

As for Fasting, you decide to voluntarily withhold from eating for several reasons such as weight loss, spiritual cleansing, body rest, and other distinct reasons.

Fasting can go on for a few hours, days, and weeks. You have actually been fasting every day of your life, yet you've never realized it.

Think about it, every night when you come home from work you eat dinner; you don't eat until the next morning. Well, you've just spent 12 to 14 hours fasting. See how easy it is?

It's no wonder the term breakfast exists. It refers to breaking a fast "break fast." It is a part of everyday, normal life.

However, for some strange reason, we have entirely overlooked its awesome power and ignored its therapeutic potential.

In plain language, fasting simply allows the body to burn off excess body fat. When you don't eat, your body uses its stored food to fabricate energy. Thus, burning fat!

Our bodies are designed to use its stored fat, that's what it's there for. So, there is nothing wrong with fasting. It's the most natural thing you can do to help your body restore balance or essentially lose weight.

Since we are constantly eating, because society tells us that it is the normal thing to do, our bodies are regularly using incoming food as energy. It never gets the chance to use up its stored energy source.

In the end, it never gets to burn any of the fat that it has stored up for when it hasn't got any incoming food to burn — it only stores and stores and stores more fat.

Typical diets do not offer the uniquely significant advantages that fasting procures.

It is free and straightforward, it saves time, and it is readily available and is scientifically proven to work.

Top tips to efficiently do intermittent fasting

- Drink plenty of water.
- Drink coffee, tea (no sugar or milk).
- Stay busy.
- Don't tell anybody you are fasting, unless you are sure that they will be supportive.
- You can try a day or 2 of fasting right after a Carb Re-fill day.
- Try On & Off fasting for at least 1 month.
- Follow a low-carb diet between fasting periods. It will increase your weight loss process and help control your cravings on fasting days.
- Don't binge after fasting.

Don't diet; change your habits

Chapter 9

Leptin the hunger usher

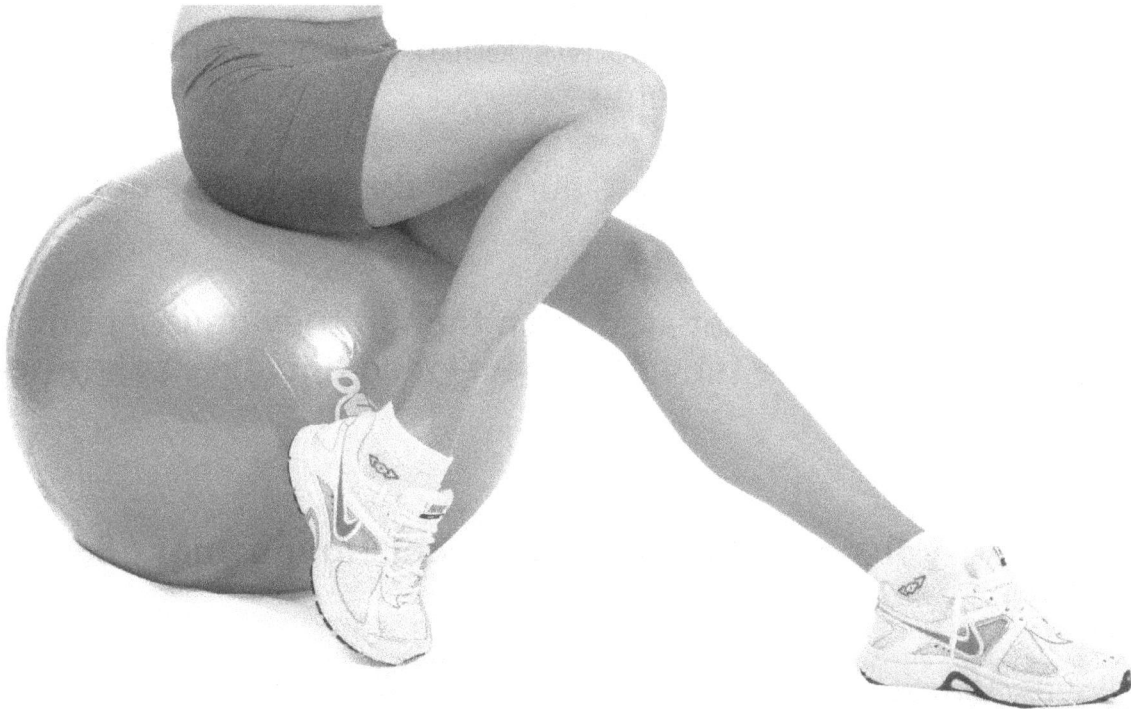

Leptin is a protein made by fat cells to control energy levels.

It regulates metabolism and appetite — as leptin levels rise, appetite diminishes, and metabolic rate increases.

This hormone does its job by telling the brain when you are full.

When leptin is released, the feeling of hunger magically goes away; when leptin levels are low, you guessed it, the body starts to cry famine; however, for many and more specifically for obese people, the problem is that the brain does not receive the release of leptin, and the signal of being "full" is not triggered.
If you want to control your body weight better, leptin regulating is especially essential. To curb your hunger, you must learn how to stimulate a leptin response in your body.

Re-stimulate your body to leptin hormones

Make those fat cells workout.

If you want to improve your body's leptin response, then only losing weight will **not** fix your problem.

You'll need to do exercises that burn off **as many fat cells as you can.**

Obese people rarely feel satiated even though they have leptin in their system. That is because they have developed a leptin **resistance**, via their fat cells.

Every day you should do some cardiovascular & aerobic exercises.

Cardiovascular exercises are workouts that increase oxygen intake, as for aerobics, they increase blood flow. They complement each other perfectly.

Simply walking 30 minutes every day can also burn enough fat to trigger a leptin response. But, ideally, a high level of **sustained activity** that increases oxygen intake and blood flow is what you should aim for.

- As you burn fat cells, stored leptin gets released.
- The overall amount of active leptin receptors gets released with this type of exercise.
- Cardiovascular exercises also boost your metabolism, so you burn fat, faster.
- You should know that your max heart rate when exercising is roughly 220 minus your age (so if you're 38, 220 - 38 = 182 beats per minute). For best cardiovascular training results, you can exercise up to 80% of your max heart rate.

- How can you monitor your heart rate? With a unique wristwatch heart monitor or Fitbit (look it up)

Every day you should perform weight resistance exercises.
Apart from strengthening your muscles, lifting weights regularly burns off fat cells and calories. The wonderful thing about exercise is that the more muscles you'll have, the easier you will burn off fat cells and release leptin into the system, **even at rest**.

Short burst HIIT are tremendously effective.

HIIT is not a typo; it means "High-Intensity Interval Training." It is a form of anaerobic exercise that consists of performing short bursts of workout at maximum intensity, blended with periods of rest or movements that are less intense to help you recover.

- HIIT encourages the natural release of **Human Growth Hormone** (HGH), which helps with fat burning and the control of leptin.
- Some of the trendiest HIIT workouts are CrossFit, Fartlek, and the 7-Minute Workout.

You can look them all up on Youtube.

Dark-colored fruits and vegetables are your allies.

Fruits and vegetables that have dark skins are an excellent source of carotenoids and flavonoids, which are **anti-inflammatory** agents that help reduce oxidation in the body and increases levels of leptin.

- Broccoli, spinach, carrots, tomatoes, winter squash, and papaya are but a few excellent sources of carotenoids.
- Pomegranate, green tea, blueberries, cherries, citrus fruits, onions, and dark chocolate are all excellent sources of flavonoids.

Why should you increase your omega-3 fatty acid intake?

For the proper functioning of the brain and body, Omega-3 fatty acids are essential.

They promote healing and decrease inflammation.

They are particularly beneficial for neurological development and its functions.

- Omega-3 fatty acids reduce blood vessel inflammation, which improves the body's capability to respond to leptin.

- Vegetable oils provided by canola, soybean, flaxseed, and fish oils, fatty fish, green and leafy vegetables, nuts, and beans, are all a selected food source of omega-3 fatty acids.

- The recommended weekly intake of omega-3 fatty acid is equal to eating at least 2 to 3 servings of 2-3 ounces of fatty fish such as Salmon, trout, mackerel, and sardines.

If you are vegan or vegetarian, then ground flaxseeds, walnuts, seaweeds, hemp seeds, edamame, and kidney beans are your friend.

Here are a few symptoms you may encounter if your body is lacking in Omega-3 fatty acids.

- Difficulty concentrating
- Dry hair, skin, and nails
- Mood swings, irritability
- Fatigue
- Poor sleep quality
- Joint discomfort and pain

Natural is more nutritious.

Most processed food lack the necessary nutrients and properties that the body requires, resulting in a faulty leptin response.

- Use natural herbs and spices that will add a kick to your meals such as sage, thyme, and basil instead of chemically filled artificial flavored foods.

Less is better.

Triglycerides(fats) are another critical culprit to leptin resistance as they hinder the carriage of leptin through the blood-brain barrier. To increase leptin sensitivity, decrease your intake of unhealthy fat.

- You can lower triglycerides by maintaining a healthy weight, **limiting fat and sugar consumption**, maintaining an active lifestyle, not smoking, and limiting alcohol.
- Genetics can contribute to having elevated levels of triglycerides.
- Some medications can also cause triglyceride levels to be high.
- Supplements of Niacin or vitamin B 3 can reduce triglyceride levels.

Sleep well.

Getting adequate sleep is essential to any weight loss regiment as it helps to regulate leptin levels. You must get at least 7 to 9 hours of good quality sleep each night.

Stay hydrated.

Staying hydrated not only helps the body absorbs nutrients and vitamins; it is also crucial in the digestion process, it influences temperament and controls hunger.

That being said, constant dehydration is likely to severely impede your sensitivity to leptin and increase your resistance to it.
To reverse this is easy, stay hydrated.

- Drink at least eight to ten cups of water, or 64 to 80 ounces, every day
- Avoid alcohol and beverages with caffeine as they actually contribute to your dehydration

Supplements are complements.

Many online supplements claim to increase your leptin levels. These are deceiving because leptin cannot enter the bloodstream and so it can't be taken as a supplement.

However, some supplements encourage leptin sensitivity and/or decreases leptin resistance.
- Irvingia is a supplement made from mango extract that can improve leptin sensitivity, among other beneficial effects
- Antioxidants can be taken as supplements such as Taurine and Acetyl L-Carnitine supplements to help decrease leptin resistance
- Grapes, blueberries, nuts, dark green veggies, and sweet potatoes are all some natural sources of antioxidants that help with leptin sensitivity

Avoid smoking and excessive alcohol consumption.

Studies seem to indicate that smoking and alcohol consumption can constrain leptin secretion. It is also evident that alcohol is extremely high in calories.

Now that you understand how **Leptin** has an enormous influence on your ability to feel full or not, and how Leptin is stored within the fat cells, we can now move on.

Chapter 10

Water is life

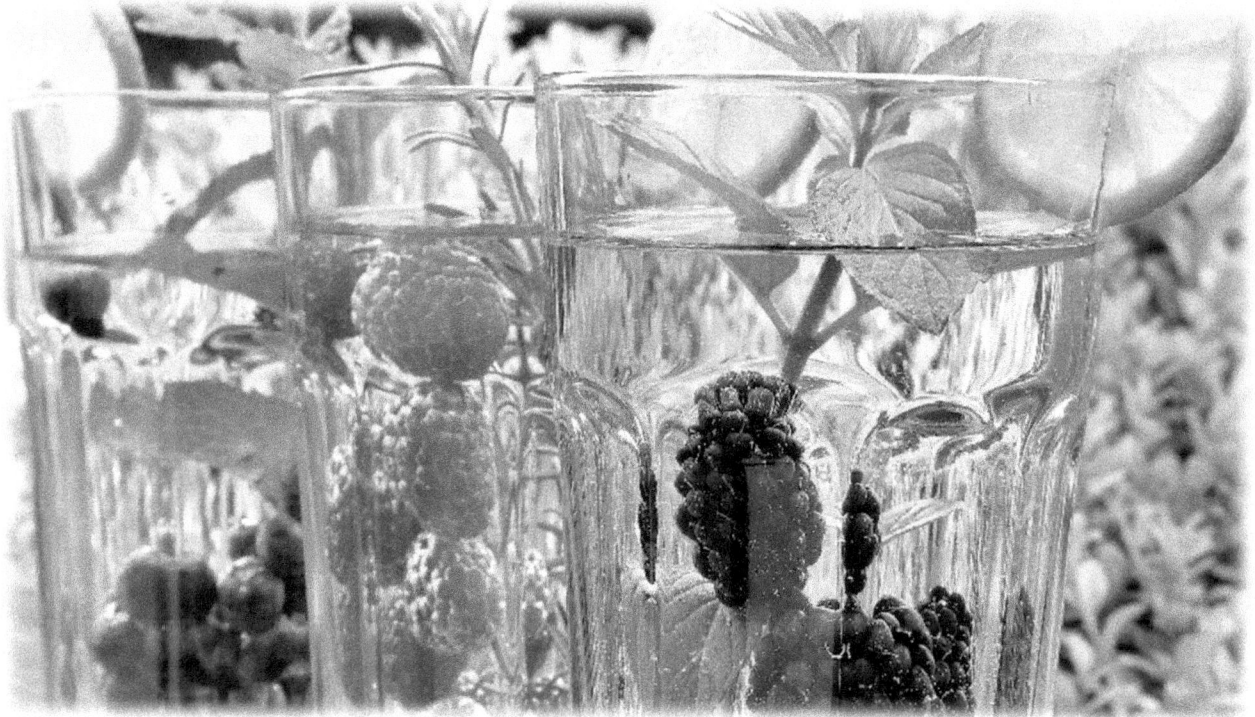

While drinking an occasional glass of red wine has some beneficial effects on the body. It is best to avoid all alcohol base drinks because of their exceedingly high-calorie content.

Almost all the fluids you consume should be only water, at least while you're in the process of losing weight.

Keep in mind that 1 of the easiest ways to get fat is by drinking your calories.

So, at all costs, avoid sodas, commercially sold fruit juices, sports drinks, calorie dense smoothies, etc.

You only need water!

And you should drink lots of it.

However, herbal teas and especially Matcha, green tea, and oolong tea are an excellent alternative for people who have a tough time drinking plain water.

It is obvious that you must not add any cream, milk, or sugar. On the other hand, Stevia, a sugar substitute that comes from a plant, and has no calories, is a rather good substitute.

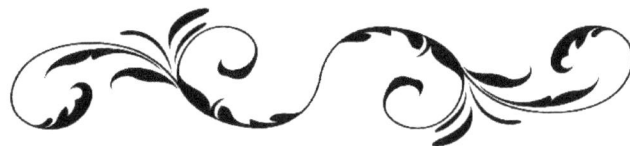

Countless reasons why you should drink plenty of water...

As reported by the editorial staff at WebMD, drinking ice cold water helps boost your metabolism because your body must work harder to warm the water up, therefore burning more calories and helping you to lose weight. Then again, that is part of the old school frame of thinking.

According to Ayurvedic medicine, the modern viewpoint of medicine, drinking warm water is less of a shock for the body. Most importantly, drinking very warm water in the morning, and regularly throughout the day, can heal our bodies, giving us more digestive power, and flushing out metabolic waste and toxins. This, in turn, helps us have a stronger immune system.

- Warm lemon water or green tea in the morning are the drinks that should replace your cold water, juice, or coffee.
- Warm water cleanses digestion by flushing out toxins and helps break down foods even faster, making it easier to digest. Conversely, drinking cold water before, during, or after you eat, can harden the oils contained in the food and leave fat deposits in the intestines.
- Water aids with constipation. Drinking very warm water in the morning on an empty stomach can help improve bowel movements and break down foods as they pass through the digestive tract.
- Warm water can alleviate pain from menstruation to headaches. It also increases blood flow to the skin and helps relax cramped muscles.
- The perfect complement to losing weight is warm water as it increases body temperature, which therefore increases the metabolic rate.
- You want to boost your body's metabolic rate every which way you can since this will helps you burn more calories throughout the

day. It is also beneficial for your gastrointestinal tracts as well as for your kidney functions.

- It improves blood circulation by flushing out the toxins that are circulating throughout the body and then enhances blood circulation.
- You'll love this one, drinking warm water stops premature aging by cleansing the body from toxins, while repairing skin cells to increase elasticity.
- It reduces your appetite; any time you feel like snacking, drink a glass or 2 of water, and you'll feel full and be less likely to snack.
- Your body needs water to **metabolize fat**. It's part of the fat burning process.
- It keeps you hydrated and healthy.
- Water helps your muscles work at their best and boosts brain functions.
- By drinking regularly, you'll be less prone to getting dehydrated while exercising.

You should drink enough water daily.

What is enough? 64 ounces or eight glasses of water is the bases of what a person should drink per day. On the other hand, if you workout a lot, you may want to triple that.

Overweight people should drink half their weight in ounces. So, if someone weighs 200 pounds, they should generally drink 100 ounces of water per day, that is about 12 tall glasses of 8oz per day.

If you're thirsty, drink! Don't delay.

Here's a shocker for you.

Your basal metabolic rate, which keeps your organs functioning, burns as much as 70% of your calories, physical activity adds about 20% and digestion about 10%.

That is a good reason why keeping your body's organs in tip-top shape by drinking water is important when wanting to lose weight.

Chapter 11

Get your beauty sleep

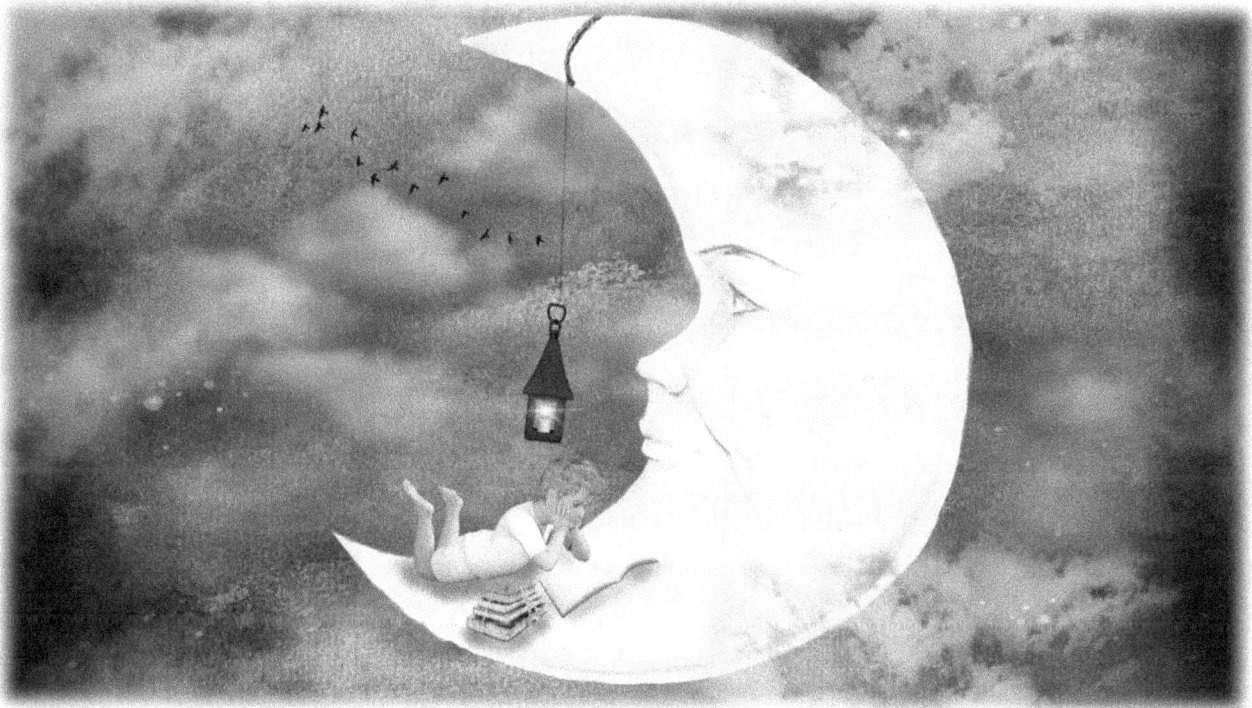

People who want to lose weight don't usually grasp how crucial it is to get enough quality sleep.

When your body lacks sleep, stress takes over your system, and your body then releases a hormone called **cortisol**. This hormone indirectly leads to **weight gain**.

It is primordial for people to realize that being constantly **deprived** of sleep will eventually take a toll on their health.

Research has proven that people who do not sleep enough or don't have quality sleep, eat more, feel hungry most of the time, and generally consume up to 350 calories more than required.

That is to say, those who stay awake late often find themselves consuming snacks and heavy meals.

If you don't get enough sleep, your body's insulin sensitivity and glucose tolerance levels will drop. This is a bad thing since your body will go into **fat storage mode** instead of being in *fat burning mode*.

When your insulin sensitivity is down, you store much more fat, which means you will **gain weight**. The same applies to glucose tolerance.

The body's stress hormone, cortisol, is increased whenever you lack sleep. This phenomenon decreases the body's ability to burn fat, and in a worst-case scenario, it can **entirely stop**.

Daily training and eating in a caloric deficit way stresses your body out, so you need sleep to rest and let your body repair itself, not to mention that you must give it time to de-stress.

"Beauty sleep" is much more then a simple expression.

All the best effort in the world to lose weight will be totally useless if you don't get enough sleep at night.

Eight hours of sleep is the basic amount you need to be at optimal health. A lot of people claim to get by on less, but at a price to their health.

As for working out before bedtime, that is debatable. A 2011 study determined that subjects slept just as well on nights when they exercised for 35 minutes right before bed as they did on nights when they didn't exercise.

If you feel too overly stimulated by exercising late at night, simply do it a few hours before bed. That way, your body temperature will return to its usual 98.6 degrees, your heartbeat will return to its resting state, and your adrenaline levels will stabilize so you can get a good night's sleep.

What's more, another research conducted in 2013 by the National Sleep Foundation's "Sleep in America" poll, did a study on 1000 people and showed that a whopping 83% of people who exercised at any time day or night, reported sleeping better at night.

Nevertheless, in case you do have some trouble falling asleep try a few of the following: Meditating or reading a book or do some light breathing exercises to free your mind from the daily stresses of life.

Stop watching late night TV.

Take note that to get a better night's sleep, it is also recommended to avoid the use of a computer, tablet, or iPhone 1 to 2 hours before bed.

If you genuinely must use such a device, try setting the screen density to a yellow tint. That will cut off most of the blue light which prevents distinct photoreceptor cells in the eye from triggering the release of a sleep hormone.

The same goes for the lighting in the room that you are in. Go for a dimmed or yellowish lighting, instead of bright white lights.

At any time, but especially on a weight loss journey, try not to burn the candle at both ends. Extreme fatigue is detrimental to weight loss.

The power of a good night's sleep should never be underestimated.

Chapter 12

Micro exercise is better than zero exercise

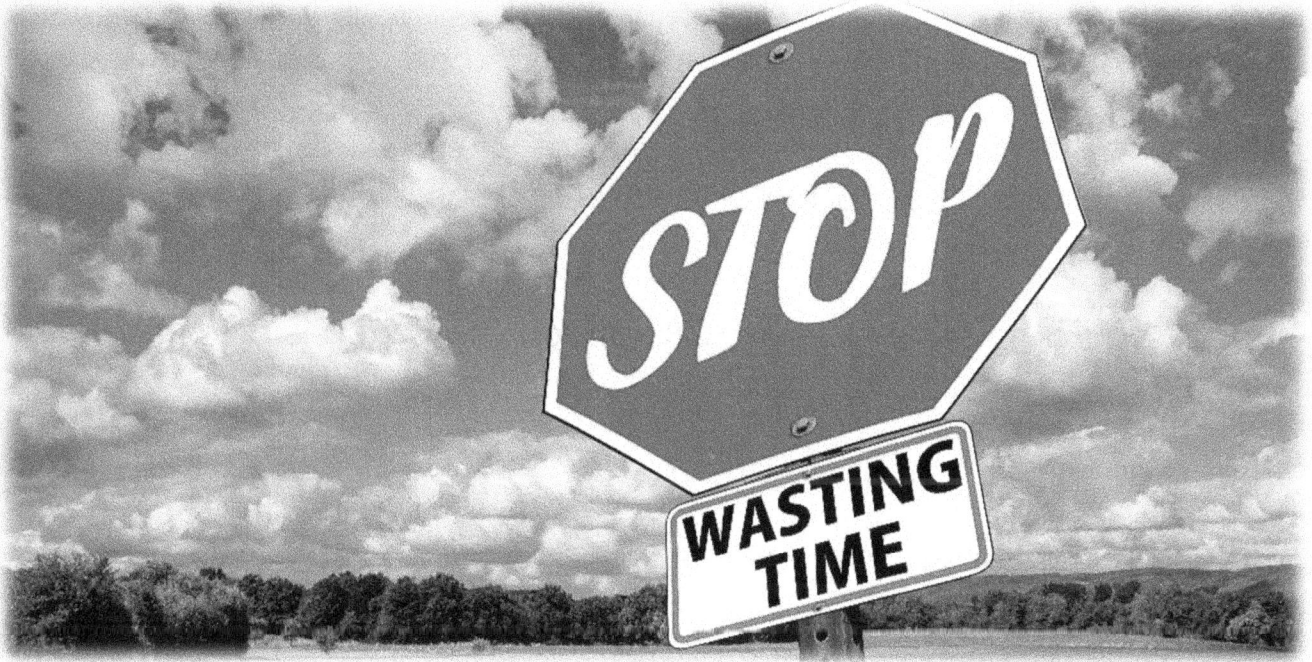

If you are like most women, you are hard-pressed for time.

You could be the mother of a newly born child who needs your full attention. Maybe you're a professional with demanding deadlines, and you still need to juggle your responsibilities as a wife and mother.

We live in a fast-paced world. Time is a precious commodity that never seems to be enough.

So, what are you supposed to then?

Well, you have to learn to improvise, use your imagination.

You may believe you are short for time, but trust me when I say that you can always manage to squeeze a little bit of physical activity somewhere. Moreover, a little bit of physical activity is by far better than none at all and I will show you a way to get your metabolism cranked up to have it burn calories all day, and all you'll need for that is a few minutes of exercise.

Let me put things in perspective.

Think about this a little, since an hour workout represents only 4% of a day, imagine what a 15-minute workout represents.

1%, yes, that's it, a 15-minute workout represents only 1% of your day!

Surely you can afford to spend 1% of your day exercising, right?

Ok, ok, if 15-minute is still too much then go for an 8-minute workout, that is a measly ½% of your day!

But what can you achieve in 8 minutes? Quite a lot!!!

Anybody no matter how busy they are can squeeze in 8 minutes.

What? Eight minutes is still too much!?!

How about 4 minutes?

Yes, yes, only 4 minutes of Tabata protocol can do miracles. Simply Google it and watch a few videos, you'll see that it's quite simple yet very effective.

The goal here is to boost your metabolic body rate within 4 minutes and cause it to be in a fat burning state for hours on end.

Is it easy to do? Of course not! But it **will** be effective.

Think about it... 4 minutes is gone pretty fast. It's a ¼% of your day!

Just imagine, you could complete a workout within a commercial break!

It's that fast!

The difference between a 1-hour long workout and a short burst of 4-minute workout is the shorter the workouts; the more intense they have to be.

There are also other tricks you can do to ensure that you burn more calories.

For example, you can get yourself a pair of ankle weights and wear them throughout the day.

You will burn more calories when you walk and move.

If you're a stay-at-home-mom, get a backpack and add some weights in it. Anything will do, put a couple of pairs of heavy shoes, a phone book or 2, etc.

The added weight will make everything more challenging, and you will burn more calories because of the added resistance.

Furthermore, you should get yourself a **Fitbit** which will track the number of steps you take daily. Aim to increase the number of steps by 100 **every day**.

Likewise, you could climb the stairs instead of using the elevator. Moreover, you could walk to the supermarket if you can.

Are you the mother of a newborn baby? Get an infant sling and place your baby in it. Then go for a 30-minute walk. An excellent exercise for you and the baby gets a breath of fresh air too.

By incorporating a few new practices and changes in your life, you will burn a lot more calories and lose weight twice as fast.

Once you have that done, get a **journal** and record your **activities**.

Chapter 13

Shaping up

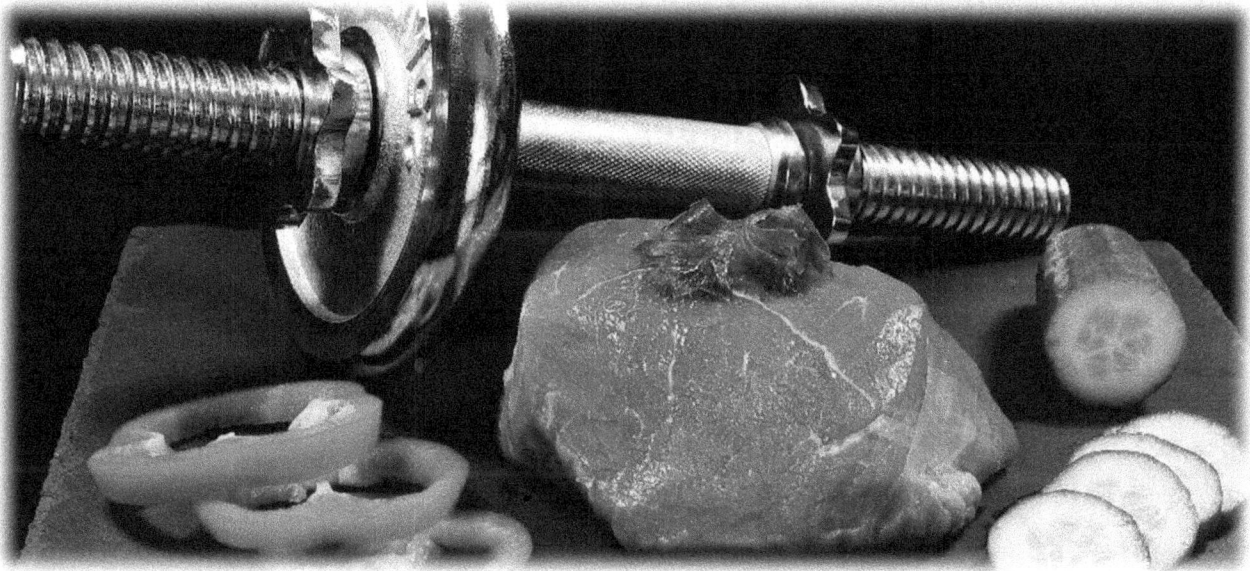

The importance of following a proper training regimen that not only boosts your stamina but also strengthens and tones your body cannot be overemphasized.

To lose weight, cardio is a fantastic way to burn calories.

Unfortunately, millions of women around the world focus ONLY on cardio workouts.

This is a **mistake** because strength training is **crucial** for weight loss too.

Remember this: The leaner muscle mass your body has, the more calories it burns **while at rest**.

That essentially means you'll be a fat burning machine throughout the day.

The best way to structure your workout will be to have 3 cardio sessions a week and 2 resistance training sessions.

The power of fasted cardio

First thing in the morning, when you still have an empty stomach, that is the most effective time to do your cardio.

Unfortunately, the notion of a strenuous workout so early in the morning does not bode well with most people.

But I have good news for you because it does NOT have to be exhausting.

In fact, it's best to keep things relatively **light**.

One of the best ways of losing weight is to go for a brisk walk first thing in the morning. A short 20 to 30-minute walk is ideal.

Something to note is that you should be able to hold a conversation while walking. You shouldn't be exerting yourself to a point where you're panting and gasping.

Remember that we're not aiming for high intensity here.

When you wake up in the morning, your body is in a fasted state. Your glycogen levels are low, and the food in your body is digested.

This means that your body will be **forced** to burn fat for fuel while you walk. It can burn up to 20% more than it would otherwise burn if you did not do a fasting morning walk.

So, during the 20 to 30 minutes that you're walking, your body is burning its fat stores for fuel.

This is an immensely potent method, and because it is not demanding, you can easily do it on a daily basis.

This morning stride will also boost your metabolic rate, and once again you'll burn calories the whole day through.

If you don't wish to walk, you may swim or use a stationary bike.

As long as it's a cardio activity that's at a **moderate pace,** your body will burn fat, and your efforts will pay off.

On the other hand, you may wish to engage in strength training or a short high-intensity interval training later in the day.

That's perfectly fine because the morning workout is just meant to speed up the fat burning process.

It's an **additional technique** to help you reach your weight goal faster. This is such an easy method that any non-disabled person can do it.

If all you can manage is a 10-minute walk, then just do 10 minutes. With time, you can slowly progress to 20 or 30 minutes.

There's really no need to go above 30 minutes.

Try it out, tomorrow morning, go for that morning walk, you'll feel the benefits right away, and you'll see the difference within a few short weeks.

Weight training

One assumption that is spread out throughout many groups of women is that they will get bulky and masculine looking if they start to train with weights. This could not be more wrong.

If they only knew how men must struggle to gain that muscular built. The advantage for women to train with weights is to look leaner and more defined.

You can cast aside all worries about looking like a female bodybuilder.

Bodyweight training such as squats, push-ups, lunges, dips, and pull-ups are great ways to work your muscles and joints.

It's crucial to work your muscles, or they will **atrophy** with age.

Look for exercises that tone your thighs, butt, and arms.

These are common problem areas for many women.

To look fit, healthy, and radiant, strength training is the curve making solution, whereas cardio will help you shed the fat.

A short 10 to 15-minute full body workout done early in the day will work miracles. This type of workout is known as HIIT...

High-Intensity Interval Training.

Here's the kicker. You can even do a HIIT workout in one spot and still sweat like crazy.

For example, let's look at this workout circuit.

1. Sit Ups – 45 seconds
2. Burpees – 45 seconds
3. Jump Squats – 45 seconds
4. Push Ups – 45 seconds
5. High Knees – 45 seconds
6. Jumping Jacks – 45 seconds
7. Burpees – 45 seconds
8. Alternating Lung Jumps – 45 seconds
9. Sit-ups – 45 seconds
10. Push Ups – 45 seconds

Between each exercise, you need to rest for 15 seconds.

You could do this workout in a cubicle. It takes up that little space.

What to remember is that you need to go as **hard** as you can go.

There is no taking it easy.

If all you have is 10 minutes, then it MUST be a **hard 10 minutes**.

The good news is that this is just 10 minutes.

If you do this workout early in the day, your body will be in fat burning mode throughout the day because of the intensity.

It creates a situation in your body, known as post-exercise oxygen consumption. That means your body will be burning calories at an **accelerated** rate for 10 to even 14 hours after your workout is over.

It's amazing what just 10 minutes can do.

The reason you do it early in the day is that your metabolism drops the moment you go to bed. This means that it is burning very little fat.

By completing your training early in the day, you'll reap maximum rewards.

It's also worth noting that it's best that you make these short workouts **full body workouts**.

Do compound movements such as squats, jumps, push ups, etc.

By recruiting as many muscles in your body as you can, you'll be ensuring that your workout is engaging the whole body.

Even 3 of these short workouts a week will transform your body within a month.

Go ahead and try them. You will be amazed.

Do remember to have 2 rest days a week.

You can split them up, or you can have both days back to back. It's really up to you.

It is very important that every week you do take a break because your muscles and nervous system need to have some recovery time.

If you go too long and hard without rest, you will stress your body out, and it will get drained out.

This is also dangerous for you to hit a weight loss plateau. If that happens, you'll be forced to take 4 to 5 days of rest to recover.

This will inevitably slow down your progress, and you might even gain some weight.

So remember to take a 2 day break every week.

Do your research online and find the best **resistance training** and **cardio workouts for you.**

Vary your workouts and challenge your body.

You'll get stronger and leaner in no time at all.

Making it fun is necessary

Make your exercise sessions fun.

Find a workout buddy if you are more consistent and motivated with one.

Don't do the same workouts daily. Monotony can discourage even the most enthusiastic person.

Try something new. Maybe yoga at the gym or kickboxing.

You could try rock-climbing too!

Feel like dancing? Check out Shaun T's workouts or Zumba sessions and follow along.

Dance while you clean the house!

The key here is to keep moving. Your caloric deficit will cause weight loss no matter what you do.

The exercise is just to speed up the process.

Do whatever you like; cycling, running, swimming.

What matters is that you MOVE daily.

A sedentary lifestyle is what causes **obesity**.

Keep moving and keep it fun!

Don't diet; change your habits

Chapter 14

Dealing with slip-ups

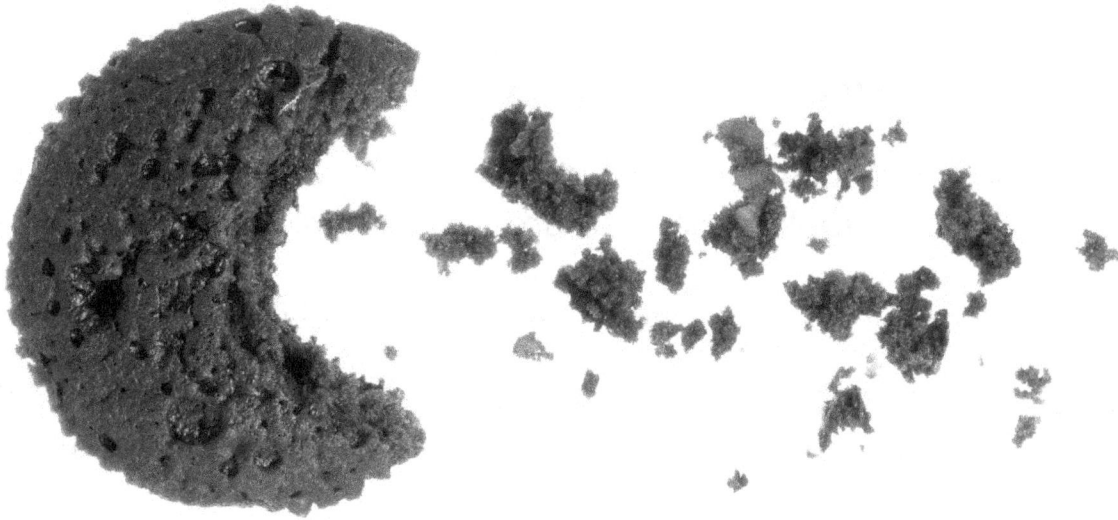

If you're like most women, sooner or later, you're going to slip-up.

You're going to go out with friends and splurge, or you're going to eat that pizza that your family has been crying out for. That's ok, you are human, and slip-ups are a part of life.

Maybe you'll even neglect a workout. Again, it happens to the best of us.

How you proceed from a slip-up makes all the difference to whether you succeed in your weight loss journey or fail miserably.

Let's look at slipping-ups with your diet first.

When you go on a weight loss journey, it usually involves eating less than you're accustomed to, to create a caloric deficit.

You'll also need to focus on eating foods that are healthy and wholesome while avoiding processed and junk food.

However, the body is already used to eating without much thought, and you're probably addicted to processed and junk food without even realizing it. Millions of people are, and when they try to ditch these unhealthy foods, they get cravings and mood swings.

The key point is to make the changes **gradually**.

Only aim for a 500-calorie deficit daily. This is a reasonable amount, and you will not be feeling like you are starving yourself.

You may feel a little peckish, but it will be manageable.

Oppositely, if you cut your calories too drastically, you will be feeling hungry all the time, and this is sheer mental and physical torture.

Your body is not used to it.

Aim to gradually reduce the consumption of harmful foods first and replace them with good ones.

If you drink 3 cans of soda daily, cut it down to 2 for a week and then bring it down to one can… and finally, put an end to the soda habit. Don't just give up sodas overnight. You'll go crazy!

Problems arise when people try to do too much too soon. They make things so challenging that compliance becomes a nightmare. People aim for perfection.

Eventually, they lose the battle of wills within themselves and give-in by eating that double cheeseburger and fries, they'll maybe even throw in a chocolate shake with that.

Guilt evades them, and they think they have failed. In fact, they may throw in the towel, believing that they are meant to be fat.

This is something that happens to millions of people.

But what anyone should keep in mind if they slip-up is that they made a single mistake.

If YOU slip-up, you have NOT failed! The only way to fail is to give up altogether, but why would you do that when you have gone so far already, and you have so much to gain by losing weight.

Simply acknowledge your slip-up and move on.

Tell yourself that you will be more mindful of what you eat.

You can easily do some "Intermittent Fasting" for 2 days, that'll set you back on track.

Ease up on your stringent diet and allow flexibility while maintaining a caloric deficit.

Do not deprive yourself of too much, too soon. Treat yourself to a small ice cream cone once and a while, you deserve it.

As for your workouts, the same mindset should apply.

Don't start-off with a bang working out 3 times per day doing HIIT, plus 1-hour weight training... you get the point.

Start-off with a morning walk and maybe 1 HIIT.

Likewise, if you miss a workout 1 day, make sure you do 1 the next day.

However, never ever miss more than 3 workout sessions in a row, or you'll conveniently fall off track, and it will be very tough to get back on it.

If you dread exercising, you're either pushing yourself too hard, or you're engaged in an activity that you have <u>no interest in</u>.

That is why it is SO important that you find workouts that are fun and engaging.

Do your research. Simply Google "best cardio workout" "best toning workouts" "Best abs workout" …

Exercises are meant to **boost** your metabolic rate and increase fat burning. But what you eat, and the caloric deficit is what really matters when it comes to fat loss.

Missed workouts and diet mistakes are **not** the end of the world and should definitely not be the end of your weight loss journey.

Stay focused but don't be so hard on yourself if you slip-up. Just do your best not to do it again.

It is a journey, and it's inevitable that now and then you get lost and hit a few bumps along the way.

If you stay on track and keep going despite your setbacks, you will reach your goal.

That's always how most people reach their goals.

Keep your chin up and keep moving forward.

Be proud of your achievements

It is totally normal to feel like giving up sometimes.

Ease up on yourself, relax, and enjoy the process.

Be proud with even a pound of weight loss.

If you knew what a pound of fat looked like, you would be delighted about having lost so much. Besides, next week you will lose more!

What matters is that you know that you'll get there, and you **must** stay positive.

Don't obsess over your weight.

Maintain the caloric deficit, do your workouts, drink enough water, get enough sleep, make your workouts fun… and relax.

You will reach your goal.

Keep your eyes on the goal, stay positive, and grateful for your accomplishments, and keep going!

Visualize where you want to be… and you'll get there.

Chapter 15

Hunger that is not real

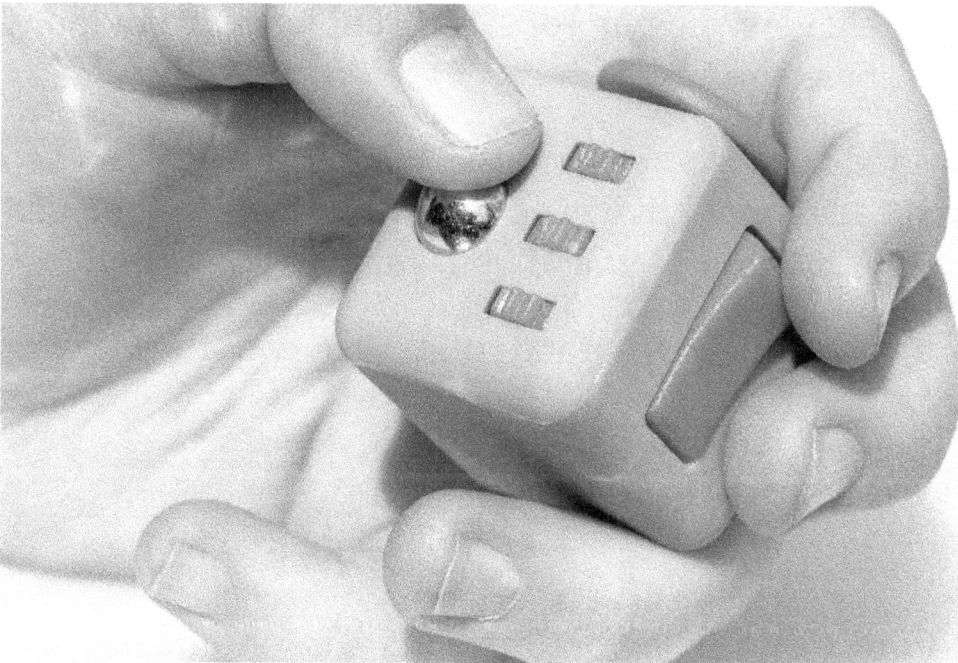

Are you an emotional eater?

"Emotional eating is when you eat in response to feelings rather than hunger, usually as a way to suppress or relieve negative emotions.

Stress, anxiety, sadness, boredom, anger, loneliness, relationship problems, and poor self-esteem can all trigger emotional eating.

When emotions determine your eating habits rather than your stomach, it can quickly lead to overeating, weight gain, and guilt."

Aug. 4, 2010 Source: TODAY

It is estimated that as much as 75% of overeating is caused by emotions.

Hence, if like so many other women in the world, you tend to eat your emotions, then what you <u>must</u> do to manage to lose weight or never gain the life-threatening weight back, is to find <u>alternative ways</u> to fill the void or tame your anxiety.

Many turn to food to relieve stress or cope with unpleasant emotions such as sadness, loneliness, or boredom.

But don't be discouraged because by practicing <u>mindful eating</u>, you can change the emotional habits that have sabotaged your diets in the past. You can regain control over both food and your feelings.

What you need are alternatives to food that you can turn to for emotional fulfillment.

Alternatives to emotional eating

- **Recognizing your hunger;** before reaching out for a bite to eat, rate your hunger on a scale of 1 to 5; 1 you are full and 5 you are famished. Make every possible effort in avoiding to eat when you are at either 1, 2, or even 3.

- **Get sufficient sleep.** As mentioned in an earlier chapter, a good night's sleep is primordial in maintaining excellent health. As a matter of fact, research shows that sleep deprivation can increase hunger by decreasing leptin levels, the appetite-regulating hormone that signals fullness. Furthermore, with adequate sleep, you'll be less tired and have more determination to fight off the urge to grab foods for comfort.

- **The 3-food delay method;** Commit first to eat 3 specific healthy foods. For example, an apple, a handful of baby carrots, and Greek yogurt. Do this before jumping on comfort foods. If after that, you still want to continue with your comfort foods, *permit yourself*. However, you will find that often, the 3 foods are plenty to satisfy your hunger.

- **Exercise regularly;** Exercising *everyday* relieves stress and puts you in a *positive mindset*, which gives you greater strength to pass on unhealthy foods. We are not necessarily talking about hard, strenuous exercise. Walking is one of the all-around best physical activity you can do.

- **Feeling depressed or lonely;** often eating is a comforting response and nothing more. In those times, when you feel sad, lonely, or insecure, call someone who always makes you feel better. Play with your pets or look at cherished pictures. Meditate. Dance to your favorite music. Watch some funny videos or movies. Do anything to make yourself laugh. That is NOT the time to sleep, because if you do, you will only wake-up with the same mindset.

- **If you're anxious;** spend your edgy energy by dancing to your favorite songs, squeezing a stress ball, or taking a brisk walk. You can also rearrange your furniture or do some cleaning. What an excellent time to organize your closet.

- **Feeling exhaustion;** treat yourself with a hot cup of Chamomile tea, take a bath, light some scented candles, or wrap yourself in a warm blanket. Listen to some soft music. Aromatherapy is also a fantastic way to relax.

- **If you're bored;** read a delightful book, watch a comedy show, explore the outdoors, take a walk or turn to an activity you enjoy (woodworking, playing the guitar, scrapbooking, sewing, crafting, etc.).

While feeling good, you should make a personal list of activities you can do instead of eating.

Because, when you feel an *abrupt* hit of hunger, that is not real hunger, it is your emotional response to some unpleasant situation or feeling in that present moment.

Something else you **can** do to break this cycle is to *take at least 5 minutes* before you give in to your cravings. That is a tremendously effective method.

In that lapse of time, try to put your finger on the trigger that caused that emotional hunger and acknowledge that it is NOT true hunger speaking. At that time, you can then choose to do 1 of the suggested alternatives to emotional eating as proposed beforehand.

To learn more on the subject read these very well-written and fascinating articles at

https://www.helpguide.org/articles/diets/emotional-eating.htm

https://www.today.com/news/are-you-emotional-eater-wbna15720217

Chapter 16

You are not Dieting; you are changing your habits

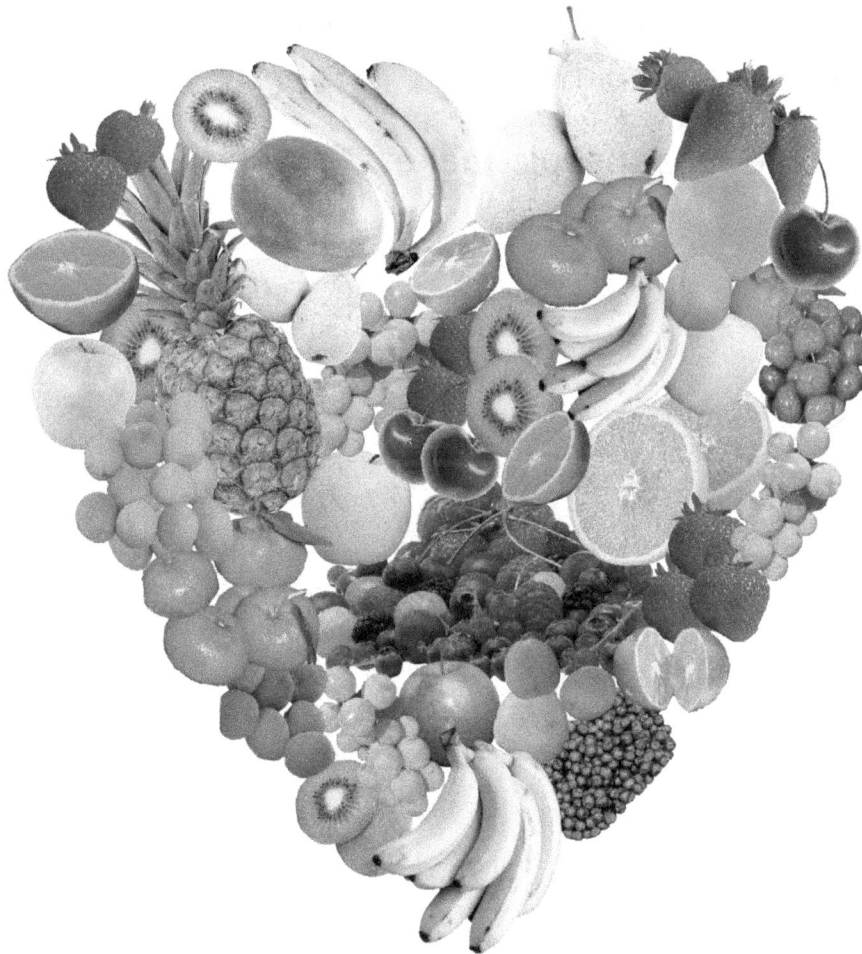

It is not surprising to know that most women who have lost a significant amount of weight, one day end up gaining it all back.

Even people on TV shows such as "The Biggest Loser" gained all the fat they had lost, once the show ended.

To stay slim, you need to change your habits, change your lifestyle.

You'll need to practice whatever you've learned in this book for **life**.

Once you reach your ideal weight, you will need to consume your calories at **maintenance** level.

This will ensure that you neither gain nor lose more weight.

Keep doing the workouts you're doing to stay fit.

It took you so much effort to get to your weight loss goal, don't lose it all by going back to your old ways.

That is the mistake most people make. But you know better now.

To resume everything in a few basic words and to see things from a clear perspective, the following is your plan.

1. Every 2 weeks, you will weigh yourself. On the same day and around the same time. (First thing in the morning or right before bed)
2. Take a front and side picture of your body, preferably in tight-fitting clothes. You will also do this every 2 weeks.
3. Note down your measurements every 2 weeks as well.
4. Eat at a caloric deficit.
5. Gradually wean off junk food.
6. Start practicing carb cycling
   o Restrict carbs near 50 to 150 grams for 3 to 6 days.
   o Refuel 1 day by eating between 225 to 325 grams of carbs
   o and eating 500 to 700 calories above MAINTENANCE level. (That is when you pleasure yourself with foods you love)
7. Then, do 1 or 2 days of On & Off fasting
8. Start the cycle again
9. Eat more protein
   o **Never consume a carb without a protein**.
   o **Never consume a fat without a protein.**
10. Do the workouts
    o Do some HIIT
11. Do fasted morning walks
12. Journal your activities
13. Journal what you eat along with its caloric and carb value
14. Drink plenty of water
15. Sleep earlier

Doesn't that seem feasible and straightforward?

Of course, it does!

Eat healthily, stay active... and be happy.

Conclusion

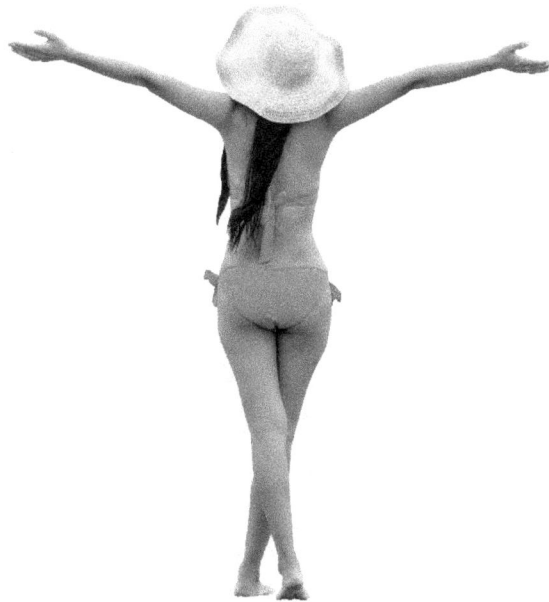

Well... you've reached the end of this health and weight loss guide.

If you follow what was stated here without giving up, you will transform your body into what you desire.

Don't quit! If you're tired of starting over... *stop giving up!*

You can do it!

Progressively change your eating habits, and soon, your unhealthy lifestyle will be a thing of the past.

Millions of women have **successfully** lost weight and kept it off.

If **they** can do it, so can you. They are not any different than you.

You have the exact same potential as they all do.

So, I wish you all the best in your weight loss journey.

Thank you

Thank you very much for taking the time to read through "Don't Diet; Change your habits".

If you enjoyed reading it and are implementing a few of the proposed recommendations, it would truly be appreciated if you could take the time to write a review.

Also, here is a special exclusive gift that I think you will enjoy...

Get the free eBook "Heal yourself" A transformative guide to better oneself and consequently improve the world we are a part of.

http://bit.ly/healyourselfreport

Likewise, if you sign-up to our newsletter, you will get a FREE 7 day Food Journal Diary to print.

Simply go to www.greatday2start.com and sign-up!

Don't diet; change your habits

As a perfect complement to this health and weight loss guide, you might enjoy the complete 90-day **Food Diary Journal + Body Measurements and Weight Tracker** by Great day 2 start, available on Amazon.

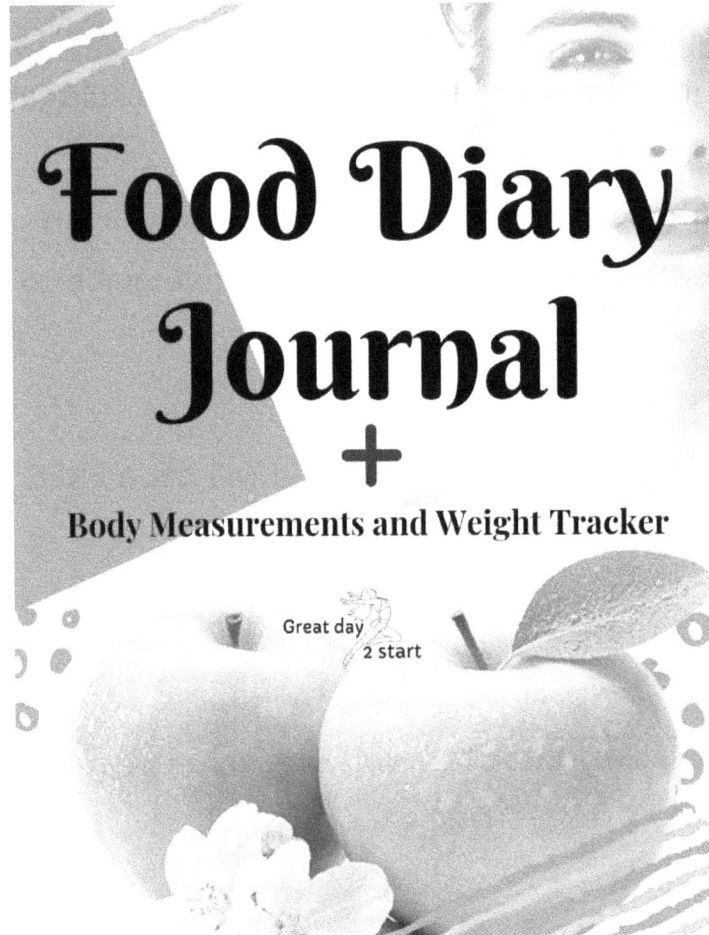

Don't diet; change your habits

We would love to receive your before and after weight loss pictures as well as your personal weight loss journey story to what@greatday2start.com

Visit us at www.greatday2start.com

Likewise, follow the author everywhere!

BookBub

https://www.bookbub.com/profile/carole-st-laurent

GoodReads

https://www.goodreads.com/author/show/16343259.Carole_St_Laurent

For health, weight loss and wellbeing of the body and soul...

https://www.facebook.com/greatday2start/

https://twitter.com/greatday2start

https://www.pinterest.com/greatday2start/

https://greatday2start.com

https://www.facebook.com/rewriteyourlifenow/

For children's books... look for books by RainbowGal

https://www.facebook.com/books.cstl/

https://twitter.com/cstlbooks

https://www.pinterest.com/cstlbooks/

http://rainbowgal.com/

or

https://carolest-laurent.com

For some romance…

https://www.facebook.com/icecreaminthesun/

Don't diet; change your habits

7-day Food Diary Journal

You can find the complete 90-day **Food Diary Journal + Body Measurements and Weight Tracker** by Great day 2 start on Amazon.

date	Meal	Food / Drink	# of Servings	Serving Size	Protein	Carbs	Sugar	Fat	Calories
				DAILY TOTALS					

date	Meal	Food / Drink	# of Servings	Serving Size	Protein (g)	Carbs (g)	Sugar (g)	Fat (g)	Calories
				DAILY TOTALS					

date	Meal	Food / Drink	# of Servings	Serving Size	Protein	Carbs	Sugar	Fat	Calories
				DAILY TOTALS					

Don't diet; change your habits

Meal	Food / Drink	# of Servings	Serving Size	Protein (g)	Carbs (g)	Sugar (g)	Fat (g)	Calories
		DAILY TOTALS						

Meal	Food / Drink	# of Servings	Serving Size	Protein	Carbs	Sugar	Fat	Calories
		DAILY TOTALS						

Meal	Food / Drink	# of Servings	Serving Size	Protein (g)	Carbs (g)	Sugar (g)	Fat (g)	Calories
		DAILY TOTALS						

Meal	Food / Drink	# of Servings	Serving Size	Protein	Carbs	Sugar	Fat	Calories
		DAILY TOTALS						

About the author

Entrepreneur, author, and founder of Greatday2start.com; a flourishing weight loss, body & soul internet wellness stop, Kina Diamond observed that the market offered an overwhelming selection of weight loss diet books.

Many of these endorsed complicated weight loss possibilities voguing between keto, paleo, vegetarian, Atkins, Mediterranean, and so many more, it's not surprising why so many folks in search of the perfect weight loss regime drown under the fat loss wave.

Consequently, what started as a personal journey to weight loss and better health, evolved into a quest to offer the perfect straightforward solution guide to healthy weight loss which could be suitable for everyone; but more precisely aimed for women.

The author thus felt compelled to offer a much simpler solution for anyone wanting to lose weight seriously, but most of all, aspiring to feel better in their bodies.

As a whole orchestra filled with strings, brass, woodwinds, percussion, and piano, is most befitting to play a beautiful classical piece, a balanced diet filled with an array of fruits and vegetables plays the role of a masterful conductor in the symphony of our health.

Kina explored, tested, and researched the trendiest diet plans and world-renowned nutritional studies related to the wellbeing of the body and mind.

The result is this effective, and easy to read guide to weight loss and better health.

www.ingramcontent.com/pod-product-compliance
Lightning Source LLC
Chambersburg PA
CBHW081656270326
41933CB00017B/3187